When Nothing Feels Predictable

When Nothing Feels Predictable:

A Path Through Cancer

Jean LeCerf Richardson, DrPH

When Nothing Feels Predictable:
A Path Through Cancer

ISBN 13

Cover artwork by Jean LeCerf Richardson
jeanrichardsonart.com

DEDICATION

This book is dedicated to the many women with ovarian cancer especially those I have met at Camp Mak-A-Dream and the Ovarian Cancer Research Alliance. The women who have survived and those who have not, continue to inspire me with their determination to live their lives with joy, purpose, faith and intelligence.

And to Jim.

"To Live Without Hope is to Cease to Live"
Fyodor Dostoyevsky

Table of Contents

FORWARD

My Fitbit log says I walked 52,077 steps last week – 23.1 miles – and 106 flights of stairs. I have passed my goal of 20 miles and set a new benchmark. Walking proves to me that I am well, and I believe it helped me to get well and to stay well, although there is not a lot of evidence to prove that.

In August 2010, I was diagnosed with Stage IV ovarian cancer. I had positive lymph nodes from neck to groin. When I was diagnosed, I had less than a 20% chance of surviving 5 years and an even smaller chance of surviving without a recurrence. But numbers are not people and nobody knows at the start how it will go. Now ten years later, I am in that small group of Stage IV exceptional responders that have never had a recurrence.

My diagnosis was in itself ironic because I had spent my career conducting cancer research. This story is about the experience of being a cancer patient with the statistics stacked against me. It is about dealing with treatment, maintaining motivation, managing hope, and thinking my way through the unknown path of cancer.

When I was diagnosed, there was nothing I wanted so much as a friend who had lived through a terrible diagnosis like mine. But I did not have that friend. I searched for a book that would share a story to guide me through treatment and give me hope, but to no avail. This is the book I couldn't find.

This book is a personal story that shares what I learned about living with and surviving cancer. I had a tremendous advantage. I understood cancer treatment from my years of research. My oncologist and my surgeon were also my colleagues. I had the advantage of trust, of familiarity, of belief in them and the treatment. Yet, I lived with the mental, emotional and physical demands common to all cancer patients. I learned ways to manage hope and to care for my body as I met the assaults of the cancer and its treatment. I was lucky, the cancer cells succumbed to the chemo and the tumor died while I survived.

This book is not a to-do list nor is it filled with fanciful solutions to serious problems. The diagnosis is a shock, chemotherapy and surgery must be endured, faith is challenged, interactions are strengthened or fractured, and beliefs about death cannot be avoided. Facing cancer is as much a mental, emotional, and spiritual challenge as it is a physical assault and a scientific puzzle.

I believe this book will be a welcome roadmap to help others facing any cancer diagnosis. All people inevitably face unexpected challenges and I hope what I share about my experience will help them walk through the dark days when they face similar challenges. This memoir is that friend that helps build understanding and resilience in facing these challenges. And beyond that, it is about recovering from these challenges and continuing to enjoy a life filled with work, friends and family, hikes and travel, good food and a mind at peace.

PART I: THE DIAGNOSIS I DIDN'T WANT TO HEAR

Jean LeCerf Richardson

Chapter 1: A Twinge, A Tweak

If someone were to ask me what I remember about the year 2010, there could only be one answer. I was diagnosed with cancer, and not a cancer that would be dealt with easily, but rather an aggressive one, Stage IV ovarian cancer which had spread throughout my lymphatic system. Cancer is an enigma. It is a person's own cells mutating and growing out of control until these errant cells overwhelm the healthy ones, and if treatment fails, cancer can destroy the entire body.

In the case of ovarian cancer this is doubly cruel. Ovaries are the source of life. How ironic that they can bracket a woman's adult life, from the confusion they cause during adolescence, to the joy of young motherhood, to quiescence and disruption during menopause, and finally, and fortunately rarely, to being a cause of illness and even death.

I spent my career, over 30 years, working at the University of Southern California School of Medicine and the Norris Comprehensive Cancer Center. My research was a broadly defined category called "cancer control" aimed at preventing cancer, and if that failed, to detecting it early and treating it optimally so that cancer patients could return to health and full functioning. But in the fall of 2010, I was not observing and studying cancer, I was experiencing cancer as a patient. I saw this disease from the other side where the excitement of research meets the terror of the disease.

*

For me, summer meant I could spend a week at art camp, and hopefully take a trip to a National Park. In July 2010, I had plans to do both. I enrolled in a woodblock printing workshop at an adult art camp, Anderson Ranch near Aspen, Colorado.

I looked forward to walking and hiking in Colorado to build my endurance so that I would go home healthier than when I arrived. The air felt clean and the mountains stood out against the blue sky as though someone had painted them also. Art camp is just as it sounds, lots of artists: professional, occasional, wannabe and first timers, most uniquely generous, warm and talented. Only the occasional person, young or old, treat camp like a competition.

I have tried almost every form of media from paint and ink, to fabric, collage, and clay. I have painted, thrown pots, sewn quilts, carved wood, bound books, and sculpted clay. I have been juried into shows, won a few awards, sold many pieces, and enjoyed experimenting without worrying about reputation or sales. Woodblock printing was new to me although it is one of the oldest techniques for printmaking.

I rented a dorm room and bought the meal plan, happy to have the camp staff do the cooking. They prepared salads that mix grains and fruits in ways I never thought of, homemade bread, cookies warm from the oven, quiche and smoked bacon for breakfast, vegetarian lasagna, trout with almonds, and roasted vegetables with pesto.

In the woodblock class, I was carving away what would not be printed and carefully preserving the actual image which would be printed. I cut the blocks gradually, printing layers of yellow, and red and blue planning for overlaps to give green and orange. The layering of a woodblock is like building information not knowing if the final overlaps of color would result in the image I had in my mind. The layering created the final print, and when it came off the printing press at the end it could be extraordinary — or a disaster. In retrospect, it feels like a metaphor for cancer treatment.

The first morning I took a walk through the valley surrounded by peaks that I imagined would be dramatic ski runs in winter. But very quickly my sitting-at-a-desk-legs became fatigued. Then again, at 61 years of age, I assumed my neglect of exercise would take a while to reverse. "Drink water," staff told me. And I did. I was unusually thirsty in Colorado, my throat felt odd, and my skin seemed to be dry and scaly. "I need to start taking better care of myself," I thought. But the fatigue continued and even small hills seemed to get harder and not easier as the week went on. And while drinking extra water meant more trips to the bathroom, I still felt dry. It seemed peculiar but perhaps, I thought, the altitude and my lack of hiking in the previous months all contributed to my slow adjustment.

On the weekend, three of us took the gondola to the top of a peak in Snowmass planning to hike the 5 miles down on a winding ski trail to the base. As we walked high up and descended through fields of yellow and purple wildflowers, I imagined what it would be like to ski down this meandering ski trail in winter. But I was also worried as my endurance was failing. It seemed odd to tire on a downhill hike. My legs were heavy and I began to feel as if there were weights strapped to them. When we got back to the dorms, I dropped into bed and slept through dinner and through the night, and that didn't feel right either.

The studios at art camp were open 24 hours a day and often the best work was done in the middle of the night. In past years, I had used that quiet nighttime in the studio to print multiple copies of prints and set them in the drying press. But in the summer of 2010, I was in bed by nine. Still, I went home from a week at art camp rejuvenated. I had met new artist friends, learned about woodblock printing, hiked, and had not cooked one meal for an entire week.

At home and back to work, the fatigue was inconsistent and easy to ignore, But, on a short hike, I again felt the fatigue. My legs felt heavy and walking up even a mild incline was difficult. Otherwise, I felt completely fine, but I had to admit to myself that something had changed.

Probably nothing significant I thought. Yet I was trying to self-diagnose what might be wrong. Perhaps the fatigue indicated a thyroid problem and the constant thirst might indicate Type 2 diabetes. I was uneasy about it and I made an appointment for a physical with Dr. Mabel Vasquez, my primary care doctor.

I told her of the changes I had noticed recently. And though I did not want to complain or even to continue believing something was wrong, I told her about my vague and inconsistent symptoms.

"My legs are unusually tired when I walk up a hill. I feel very dry — my skin is dry; my mouth and throat are dry; I need to carry and drink water all of the time. Maybe it's Type II diabetes," I ventured, "I have that in my family."

"OK, we can test for that," she said.

"My throat feels odd, especially when I bend over or try the yoga position, downward dog. It feels like a lump in my throat sometimes, like when you feel upset. I wonder if there is something wrong with my thyroid".

"It feels normal," she said as she palpated my neck. "I could send you for an ultrasound. Maybe I just can't feel it. Let's check it out," she said.

As Mabel finished her exam she said, "You seem strong and fit. I wish all of my patients in their early 60's were doing as well."

And she was right. I was on no medications. I had no chronic or acute illnesses. I had no limitations of activity. All of my medical screenings were up-to-date, and all were normal. It seemed I was in great health.

I was reassured — this must be nothing I thought. Was age catching up with me? Is this what it felt like to be 61? But, why all of a sudden was I dragging? Shouldn't aging be a gradual decline and not an abrupt loss of energy? If it was something important, she would have found it, I reasoned. I was caught between relief and uncertainty. I wanted to believe everything was fine and yet I felt that something was wrong, a problem that just hadn't been found. With that, I headed off to the lab for blood tests and then to the radiology department to schedule the thyroid ultrasound.

My husband Jim and I had a trip planned to Zion and Yellowstone National Parks and I scheduled the ultrasound for soon after we got back.

*

A week later, Jim and I drove across the Mojave Desert, past the glitz of Las Vegas, without stopping, and on to Zion National Park. We spent a day hiking trails along the floor of the canyon with red rock cliffs surrounding us and the river, calm in summer, but still continuing to carve the canyon. From Zion, we headed for the long drive to Yellowstone to meet my brother Barry and sister-in-law Chris. It had been 20 years since we had been there a few years after the massive 1988 fire that nearly burned the Old Faithful Inn. I remembered how the vegetation was just beginning to come back then and I wondered how it would look now, years later.

Jim and I have traveled and camped with our children throughout the United States, Europe, and Great Britain and though the children are grown, married and have children of their own, we continue to explore these wilderness areas. We have hiked trails in national parks from Shenandoah to Mt Rainer and Denali. Jim even spent many years trail running in the San Gabriel Mountains, something that worried me and I had no desire to do. Although I had not camped as a child, Jim had taken many camping trips in the Sierras and had taught me some basic skills. But, on this trip we had a cabin reserved near Yellowstone Lake.

My brother, Barry's career was in publishing business journals and running large professional conferences; he is a planner of events. Jim and I were happy to have him organize day trips for all of us. We went white water rafting on the Snake River. Wet and laughing, we splashed through the rapids along with a young family and their teen-aged children riding the front of the raft as it bucked its way downstream. We hiked the rim of the Yellowstone Canyon. We kayaked on Yellowstone Lake and watched a bald eagle fly over us and land in a tree along the shoreline. It was easy to spot, the white head like a misplaced golf ball high up in the evergreens lining the lake. I lay back in my kayak and gazed at the eagle until it took off again, flying low so I could hear the powerful wings lifting and carrying it away over the lake.

We went fly-fishing with a guide who provided waders and high boots, to cross the streams. We stood in the middle to cast with the rapidly moving water nearly knocking us down. Jim, Barry, and Chris began to pull in native brown trout with barbless hooks so that they could be released unscathed. Jim had been fly fishing as a boy and still had his beautiful bamboo rod at home and I could tell he was wondering why he had let years go by since he had been fly fishing. By the middle of the day after tromping around through streams and trying to catch a fish – I hooked one but pulled in none. I was exhausted and lay down on the grassy banks nearly falling asleep, and I wondered if my low enthusiasm for fishing had sapped my energy. Perhaps it was an excuse to just enjoy looking at the sky and letting the fish swim on. I knew I was as fit as everyone else; but there was no question that on that day, I was the weak link and I did not like seeing myself that way.

A few days after coming home, I had my thyroid ultrasound. The technician put the gel on my neck and moved the ultrasound wand back and forth and up and down seeming to dwell on a particular spot. Then she said she wanted the supervising physician of diagnostic radiology to take a look also and she left the room to get him. As I waited on the exam table a shudder of anxiety passed through me. When they came back the whole procedure was repeated again.

"Your thyroid looks normal, but there is an abnormal lymph node," the doctor told me. "It's under the clavicle bone. It's bigger than it should be. I think we should do a needle biopsy. I can do it right now if you want."

I did not like the sound of an enlarged lymph node and if my thyroid looked normal then what was it? "Please, not cancer," I thought.

"Yes, do it now," I said, not expecting this but wanting to get it over with.

He inserted a needle into my neck where the lymph node was located and drew out cells that a pathologist would later examine to see if they looked cancerous. It felt more uncomfortable than painful. The cytology tech arrived and took a cursory look at the specimen under a microscope to make sure the needle biopsy had captured sufficient cells for the pathologists to make a diagnosis. As I turned to look at her, I wondered if I could tell anything from her expression. But I couldn't, her face told me nothing. And so, I would need to be patient as I continued to tell myself that it was fine — maybe just a big lymph node, certainly nothing to worry about. I put my mind on work and pushed thoughts of cancer away.

Two days later, my doctor, Mabel called. "It's cancer," she said "it's not clear what kind. The cells look like they might be thyroid or ovarian."

I was stunned and I could not find words. How could there be uncertainty over these two drastically different diagnoses? My mind swirled through the possibilities. The lymph node was in my neck. "It's got to be thyroid," I thought. And faced with cancer, I hoped it was thyroid cancer. It is most often easy to treat and the prognosis is usually good. That must be why my neck felt odd, I thought. But still, I worried. If it was thyroid cancer then why did the thyroid look normal on the ultrasound?

Forcing myself to remain calm, Mabel and I talked about the treatments for thyroid cancer. But when it came to even considering or talking about ovarian cancer, I couldn't do it. I knew ovarian cancer could be deadly and the treatment is hard. I didn't want to think about it or talk about it. "Later," I said, "if it is ovarian, we can talk about it later, not now. I don't want to think about that one." But the questions persisted. Why did my thyroid look normal? The node was in my neck. If it was ovarian cancer, that meant it had already spread.

Hoping it was all a big mistake, I asked, "What pathologist looked at the slides?"

"Dr. Sue Ellen Martin," she said.

And then I knew the results were correct. I couldn't hide behind the belief that the pathologist got it wrong, that perhaps it wasn't cancer after all. Sue Ellen and I, together with our friends Susan and Kay, went to the theater and dinner together several times a year. I knew she would not make a mistake, for me or for anyone. I thought about her examining slides with my name on them hoping she would not see cancer, but then being the first to know. I had to resist the urge to call her. I needed to let her do her job without interrogating her. I knew there would be more tests and the time would come to talk. I kept believing and praying that I had developed thyroid cancer and not ovarian cancer.

Ovarian cancer is one of those deep body cancers with ambiguous or even no early symptoms and no routine screening tests to catch it early. It is usually diagnosed late when it has already spread. The only number that came into my mind was 25%. But I couldn't remember. Was it 25% chance of survival, for one year, two years, five years or longer? And what was it for me? That was a whole different question. Though I couldn't remember the statistics, I was certain that this was bad and I knew it had been called the "silent killer" for a reason. But my symptoms were not typical of ovarian cancer. I had no bloating or abdominal pain. I did need to urinate often but I was also drinking a lot of water. I still felt fatigued and my legs felt heavy. But these symptoms were subtle, inconsistent and could be any number of different problems. Maybe that subtlety is what made the symptoms typical. They are a whisper and not a shout. I was not in pain, I was not bleeding, I was not bedridden, I was working and now, just weeks before my 62nd birthday, I felt healthy. I still had hope that maybe it was not ovarian cancer after all.

Mabel scheduled a CT scan for two days later. I was given two large bottles of contrast fluid to drink while waiting for the scan that would tell me how far the cancer had spread. As I looked around at the people in the radiology waiting room, I wondered why they were there. Did they have cancer also? I am sure I looked like a healthy woman drinking large volumes of unpleasant liquid. But the overwhelming reality was that I was trying very hard to believe I did not have cancer.

The CT scan technician recognized me from my work at the Norris Cancer Center and I recognized him as well. It was disconcerting. What was I doing at the Norris in the role of patient? I changed into a gown and lay on the scan platform with my arms above my head. The CT machine looked almost like a big white front load washing machine. The tech went into the control room and talked to me through the intercom. The platform slid in and out of the CT as different parts of my body were scanned.

Over the intercom, the technician's voice told me, "Hold your breath." I could hear the scan working. Then, "Breathe," he said.

This went on for 20 minutes. It was important not to move at all. But I couldn't help myself and I swallowed. "Don't swallow," he told me along with the instructions not to breathe. The CT made me feel claustrophobic as I lay in the metal tube. I needed to concentrate to keep myself calm. With my eyes closed, I pretended to be fine. "Just relax," I told myself, "It will be over soon." But that 20 minutes felt like an hour.

After the scan was done, I got dressed and went out of the CT room and past a glass enclosed room where several people in white coats were looking at screens. They turned to look at me and I wondered if they were looking at my scan and what they saw and what they knew.

I did not need to wait long. Mabel called the next day. "Yes, it is cancer," she said.

I pressed her for more information, "Where is it, where is the primary site? Where did it start?"

"I'm not sure yet," she said.

"Well, where can you see it?" I asked.

"It has spread," she said hesitating. When I pushed her for more information, she told me, "You have malignant lymph nodes in your groin, your abdomen, your neck, your armpit, near the branching of the trachea in your chest, and the peritoneum looks thickened," she told me. "Usually, you cannot even see the peritoneum on a CT scan, but yours seems to be thickened."

The peritoneum is like a thin sack that surrounds all the organs in the belly. Why would it be thickened? Was the cancer causing this?

"Does it look like ovarian?" I asked.

"It looks almost like lymphoma on the scan," she said, "but Dr. Martin says the cells are definitely not lymphoma. From the pathology and the scan, it looks aggressive. We need more tests to pin it down. I'll arrange it and call you tomorrow."

I continued to hope that this was some other cancer that was more easily treated than ovarian. But if Sue Ellen thought it was ovarian, I had to believe her even though I still could not accept it. Would I be one of those women with a late diagnosis that goes from feeling well to dying within a few short months? My mind began to tumble; quick opposing thoughts raced by: I would be fine — this is really bad — it must be wrong — I feel healthy — I came in for a little problem and now this big problem — my life could be over — treatment is miserable — what about my kids — it has to be wrong — I must face this — and on and on it went, so fast that I knew I needed to just get off the phone

Rationally and calmly, I thanked Mabel and told her I appreciated her sending me for a further work-up even though she initially could find nothing wrong.

"I'm as surprised as you are. I didn't expect this at all. You have never been a complainer," she replied. "I really had to listen and believe you when you said something was wrong." I knew that this kind of care was not always the case and patient's complaints are not always listened to or followed up. I felt fortunate that she had trusted my concerns.

After I hung up, I told Jim. We were both in such a state of disbelief that we couldn't even cry. Sitting together on the sofa in our living room, we could not believe that cancer was now our new reality. We were both numb and mute. The wind was taken from our sails and our lungs. And just like that, I knew that my life and his life had just changed dramatically. The future was uncertain. The days ahead would be filled with hospital visits and chemotherapy and surgery. I could not believe I had cancer at all, and I especially could not believe it had spread. I had spent so many years of my career working on issues of early detection and here I was with a cancer that seemed to be everywhere. How could it be when I had no pain and such easy symptoms to ignore? I wanted to deny that it could be that bad, although, at some level, I knew that it was.

We were filled with questions that nobody could answer. How would this be treated? Was it too late? And the most important question, "Could my life be over very soon?" I was working at a career I loved, with a family and four young grandchildren I adored, and with all sorts of plans for retirement in a few years. Despite the new fatigue, I felt vibrantly healthy. I saw myself as a 61-year-old woman who skied, hiked, kayaked, rode horses and none of this squared with cancer, not any cancer, never mind one that had already spread throughout my body. All we could do was hold each other, there were no words to confront the reality, and the fear, and the disbelief.

But while my emotions were numb and unfocused, my actions were not. I was already making lists and plans. Which of the clinicians I knew would I call to get the help and treatment I would need to survive?

Chapter 2: A Thunderbolt

In 1980, I was fresh out of finishing my doctoral degree in public health from UCLA and was newly hired at the crosstown rival, the University of Southern California (USC). I had been recruited by the Norris Comprehensive Cancer Center at USC and my very first project was to develop a research proposal for a study on patient compliance with chemotherapy. A Request for Applications (RFA) had been issued by the National Cancer Institute (NCI), and the deadline was 6 weeks after I started work at USC. Like a blind date, I was introduced to a young assistant professor named Dr. Alexandra Levine who I would work with to apply for the grant.

After much discussion, planning, writing, and editing, we mailed our proposal to the NCI. Several months later, we received notification that our project was approved and funded. It was her first big NCI grant and it was mine as well. We were excited neophytes in the world of NIH funded research. As good fortune would have it, that started our career-long collaboration and our life-long friendship. We continued to work on cancer research together for the next 33 years and as the AIDS epidemic swept the world, we worked together on studies of women with HIV as well as studies of AIDS prevention and early detection and compliance with antiretroviral therapy for those already infected.

Over the years, we have supported each other through good times and bad times. We have worked as colleagues on research studies and published papers together. But we have also supported each other as friends through the deaths of her parents and mine, through professional disappointments and achievements, and through personal and professional decisions. These weighty discussions often took place as we walked the three-mile loop around the Rose Bowl and up and down hiking trails in the San Gabriel Mountains, trying to fit exercise into our busy schedules.

Alexandra is an expert in lymphoma, so I knew if it was lymphoma, she was the person I needed to talk to. I called her home and left a message. "I have cancer. There are positive lymph nodes all the way from my neck to my groin. They say it looks like lymphoma on the CT scan but Sue Ellen says the cells are definitely not lymphoma and may be ovarian. Please give me a call, I need to talk to you."

Two days later, I got a call on my answering machine. "Hi Jean – it's Alexandra. We are on vacation on a ship off the coast of Iceland right now. I just listened to playback messages from home and I heard yours. I really want to talk to you. We are seven hours later than you." In the background I heard her husband, Victor, calmly giving instructions on how I should dial to reach her on the ship off the coast of Iceland.

Amazingly when I called her back, the call went through. Despite a bad connection, she heard a few sentences and said, "you need to get a CT guided core biopsy and it has to be done by Dr. Boswell. He is the Chief of Diagnostic Radiology. He does all of the core biopsies for my patients. I'll call Mabel to order it."

I had excellent insurance and being part of the medical school faculty – I was not fighting to get my needs met. I knew what I needed and I had close friends who could guide me and help me. After 30 years at the Norris, my work place felt like home and my colleagues felt like close friends. The testing and diagnosis progressed without pause. But this is not what all patients experience. Some women experience months of dismissed symptoms and a missed or delayed diagnosis, all the while the cancer is ticking away in their bodies. I was grateful to not be in that situation.

I felt like I was operating on two separate paths. I was going to work and teaching students and going to meetings – but I was also having tests that would tell me whether I had a disease that might kill me. My mind meandered back and forth between these realities, clinging to the healthy me and then drifting to the worried and threatened me.

I had a few days wait for the core biopsy. My anxiety built as I waited for my appointment and I wasn't even sure how that biopsy would be done. The afternoon appointment a few days later started with a transvaginal ultrasound of my ovaries. Surprisingly they looked normal. But relief was quickly followed by worry. Could whatever it was and wherever it started, be even worse than ovarian cancer? Where was the primary tumor? I didn't have long to think about possibilities because the next procedure was the CT guided core biopsy.

I lay on my stomach while Dr. Boswell numbed my back and then I was slid into the CT. The CT was used to find an enlarged lymph node deep in the center, the core of my body, where the cancer had already spread. A long needle was inserted into my back to reach these lymph nodes and retrieve more cancer cells for the pathologists to look at. I reverted to my childbirth classes of over 35 years before to control my breathing, to focus, to block pain, and to maintain my ability to stay calm.

"Are you OK?" the nurse said with concern.

"Don't worry I'm just breathing," I said. It sounded like a silly answer and I didn't know if she understood what I was doing but I couldn't explain further right then and I continued my controlled breathing until it was over.

I expected to get up, get dressed, and go home. "No, said the nurse, you need to recover for a while." Instead of making my escape, I rolled over onto a gurney and was taken down the elevators to the day hospital on the first floor of the Norris for observation. I frequently took these elevators up to my office on the third floor and down to the cafeteria in the basement. But now I was a patient in the same elevator. I hoped that none of my colleagues would see me, but from the vantage point of lying on a gurney I really could not tell whom I was being pushed past. I realized right then that any intention I may have had to hide my diagnosis would need to be put aside. I had not even confronted the decisions of who to tell and how and when and in what order. My colleagues would soon know and it was futile to think otherwise.

Dr. Boswell came by to check on me as I recovered in the day hospital. I wanted to know right away what he found.

"It's definitely not lymphoma," he said. I began to ask him about other organs. I felt like the kid who keeps asking "what about this and what about that?" No, he didn't think it was pancreas cancer. No, it didn't seem to be colon cancer either. Perhaps it was renal or gynecological he said, but they wouldn't be sure until the pathologist looked at the biopsy cells. How could it not be clear by now? I felt frustrated. After biopsies and imaging, what more would be needed to figure it out?

"What about the ovaries?" I asked.

"They looked normal on the ultrasound."

"What about the peritoneum?"

"Yes, it was thickened and that is not normal. Yours looks more like sandpaper, not smooth and thin, as it should be."

I didn't quite understand this and I imagined the peritoneum with small tumors or a sprinkle or perhaps a slime of cancer cells covering it. I kept asking questions, until he finally said more tests were needed to reach a final diagnosis and to find the primary site where it all started. It would take just a bit longer.

By then it was evening, the day hospital was emptying out and the nurse seemed glad to discharge me and send me on my way.

I went home and emailed Alexandra to tell her the CT guided core biopsy was done and Dr. Boswell was certain it was not lymphoma. It was important to get the specific diagnosis correct because it determined the treatment as well as the prognosis. I could not proceed to treatment until they knew exactly what they were treating.

The next day Mabel called and told me it looked like primary peritoneal cancer. I had never heard of this diagnosis before. She explained that it is an unusual form of ovarian cancer. Ovarian cancer can occur on the ovary itself, but also less commonly in the fallopian tubes or on the peritoneum where mine seemed to have spread; but all are considered forms of ovarian cancer. The cells, the prognosis, and the treatment are the same. It is now thought that all three forms start in the fallopian tubes, and specifically in the cells at the end of the tubes that look like a flower closest to the ovary called the fimbria. Ovarian cancer usually spreads in the abdomen and can eventually invade adjacent organs such as the colon. When ovarian cancer has spread to the lymph nodes or to the liver, it is classified as Stage IV. But the pathologists wanted a biopsy of tissue from my uterus to rule out uterine cancer and so, yet another test was needed.

The gravity and dread of cancer that had already spread throughout my mind and my body and that I had never suspected, was beginning to overwhelm me. How could this be happening to me? I was filled with disbelief at the same time that the reality of each mounting piece of medical evidence told me that it was true. Alexandra sent an email from the ship off of Iceland and yet again to my amazement; I was able to receive it.

She wrote, "Aggressive" tumor can be a misleading statement...chemo works by killing cells that divide rapidly... it's like the concept of Burkitt's lymphoma...the percentage of cells dividing at one time is >99%, and that's one of the criteria for diagnosis...yet, the tumor is CURABLE over 80% of the time. Do NOT let that word cloud up your mind."

I replied, "I understand what you are saying.... I am working it through. I just want to get on with this and start treatment." Still, I was in a fog of unreality, fearful while holding it together.

A few days later I was scheduled for a uterine biopsy. Again, I had a long-term colleague, Dr. Laila Muderspach, a gynecologic oncology surgeon. I had known and worked with Laila since before her first child was born and he had just graduated from college. If there was going to be any cutting on my body, she was the person I trusted. But first, I wanted her to be the one doing the uterine biopsy.

When we met early in the morning for the uterine biopsy, she said, "I bet you are as surprised as I am to be here. Your case is somewhat unusual. Usually, women have bigger tumors in the abdomen and slower spread to the lymph nodes." I seemed to have a rapid spread to the lymph nodes but not a single big tumor in my abdomen. Instead, the cancer seemed to be in a layer coating the peritoneum. I imagined "cancer snow" covering the peritoneum.

"Unusual does not mean bad," she said. "I have seen women with cancer in the lymph nodes do very well." She told me that she had a similar patient who was now a twenty-year survivor. She was giving me hope, but we both knew how serious this was.

The results from the core biopsy were in. The cells from the core biopsy looked different from the cells from the original needle biopsy of the lymph node under my clavicle. One of the pathologists was concerned that there might be two separate primaries, but another thought they were the same primary that had rapidly mutated as it spread through my body. I was not sure which was worse, but in the end the worry was the same. There were at least two different cells in these tumors. Some of the mutated cells may be susceptible to the chemotherapy. But some may be resistant and that would be a very bad thing.

How did I go from hiking, kayaking, fishing and rafting in Yellowstone, to having a diagnosis of cancer only two weeks later? Moreover, how did this little unnoticeable lump in my neck turn out to be cancer that had started in my abdomen? And though I knew it was metastatic, how could I keep saying "it has to be early; I feel fine" when I knew better. I just couldn't say it to myself. I could not say Stage IV to myself.

Fearful images flooded me. What is Stage IV disease other than a likely predictor of death, of my death, but also a memory of my mother's death twenty years before? My mother's robust Irish face, her freckled arms reduced to bone and sagging flesh from multiple myeloma. If she felt panic or bitterness, she did not let me see that. What I saw was a mix of acceptance and frustration that occasionally erupted into anger, until the time for morphine and the end came, perhaps too long in coming.

Chapter 3: Get Ready – The Storm is Coming

A few days later, the results were in and now everyone agreed. It was definitely ovarian cancer.

When I heard the diagnosis of ovarian cancer, my immediate thoughts were a mental stew of denial, resignation, and resilience. I might not live to see another spring or another birthday. My grandchildren were young; they would not even remember me. Imagining my own death was incomprehensible. How could I imagine everyone moving on while I was cremated? Dust to dust. I was not ready to be dust. The thought of the cancer working its way through my body with so little warning was a puzzle I could not solve. Even as I tried to work out the edges and the corners to fill in the center, this picture had no meaning, it did not make sense.

Cancer is one of those diseases that often carries a burden of guilt. People newly diagnosed, and I was one of them ask, "What did I do wrong to get this disease?" In the past people have hidden the diagnosis from shame or fear. At times family members would ask physicians not to tell the patient the true diagnosis. Hiding and blaming are part of this disease. It is the blame of smokers who later develop lung cancer or women who never get mammograms and develop breast cancer. We are referred to as "cancer victims" and "blaming the victim," is a way for the well to shield themselves from feelings of their own vulnerability. It is not just the onlookers who blame; there is also the interrogation of the self, the looking for the reason and the fault that occupies the mind of the newly diagnosed. It is not the pathetic and whinny "why me and not somebody else?" because really why not me? It is simply, "Why?" It is the search for reasons or meaning when the answers are unknown.

For women with gynecologic cancers there is an inevitable association with sexuality and a wonder about what caused this to happen. Was it too much sex? Was it not enough sex? Was it too much good sex or too much bad sex? Was it birth control pills? Was it a difficult menopause? Was it the tubal ligation or the cesarean birth? Was it sexually transmitted diseases? Was it tampons? Was it an abortion? Was it too many babies or too few? Was it talcum powder? Was it breast feeding or not? It needed to be explainable and understandable even if that explanation made no sense and had no basis in scientific data. Or maybe it was all bad luck, and what do we mean by luck anyway?

I have colleagues, epidemiologists, who have studied the causes of ovarian cancer. There are confirmed scientific findings that birth control pills for at least five years, tubal ligation, having babies, and breast-feeding are all protective. Family history especially for those carrying high-risk mutations in the BRCA1 and BRCA2 genes are at increased risk. But nothing is a perfect predictor of who will or won't get this disease. These confirmed factors increase or decrease the probability but none of them are absolute predictors. In the same way that many people who smoke don't get lung cancer and not all people who develop lung cancer are smokers. Smoking increases the probability of developing lung cancer but it does not always cause it and those who do not smoke are not absolutely protected. The factors that cause the many mutations that accumulate in a cell to cause it to go from normal to abnormal, to cancer, are still largely unknown.

*

And yet I also found my resilience and my ability to confront it. I found my hope that I could survive this. Firefighters enter burning buildings when others are running out. Why do they do it? Because they care about putting out fires to protect both property and lives, but they do so with caution and only after extensive training. They know what they are doing, they evaluate their risks, they believe they have the skills to deal with the unexpected, and they have confidence that outweighs their fears. At least I think that is what is happening. Because of my background as a scientist studying cancer, some of this thinking applied to me as I was getting ready to start treatment.

Cancer cells were traveling through my lymphatic system. The lymphatic circulation travels everywhere in the body just as the blood stream does. Surgery is usually the first treatment for ovarian cancer but because it was throughout my body, that would not work in my case. The surgeon couldn't just cut it out. Chemotherapy was the only treatment that could reach the cancer throughout my entire body. When chemo is given before surgery, it is called neoadjuvant and it is being used to shrink the tumor or eradicate it so that surgery will be more effective afterwards.

Chemotherapy and lots of it, that was the initial way to fight my disease. The way I thought about chemotherapy was likely different than most people because I had conducted studies on patients undergoing chemotherapy. Was I afraid of the chemotherapy? Perhaps. But like the firemen, I rushed toward it. Chemo was the fire hose to put out the fire of cancer before my building burned down. My goal was to save the building and the people in it, and in this case, I was the only person in there, so I was trying to save myself.

My first study funded by the NCI looked at how patients with cancers of the blood cells (the leukemias and lymphomas) actually took the oral pills that were prescribed and whether they missed appointments for infused chemotherapy. We provided educational and interpersonal supportive interventions, to see whether we could improve compliance with the treatment regimen. The interventions were effective in increasing compliance with home medications and with infused chemotherapy visits and resulted in improved survival. Those lessons stuck with me as I contemplated starting chemo myself.

I wasn't sure which of the oncologists in the cancer center specialized in ovarian cancer. When I asked my friend, Dr. Darcy Spicer, who was the chairman of medical oncology, to help me decide who should be my oncologist, he immediately said, "Dr. Agustin Garcia. He trained with the best gynecologic oncologists in the country and he handles our patients with ovarian cancer." Laila, my surgeon, said he was "a gifted oncologist" and my friend Sue Ellen agreed. That settled it.

Although I had known Agustin for many years, I had never had more than a cursory conversation with him. Agustin's picture was on the Norris Cancer Hospital advertising posters, an engaging picture of a young physician sitting on a stool, smiling and talking with a bald woman in a baseball hat. They seemed to be enjoying a joke. Agustin looked very young as he does in person. Several months later when I showed my son David the picture, he looked at it and said, "How old is this guy?" "Hard to tell," was my answer, "somewhere in his forties I think, don't worry, he has been at this for a while." I could tell he might have liked a sage looking grey haired physician rather than someone who looked only a few years older than he was.

A few days later I was in my office trying to concentrate on work while knowing that my first appointment with Agustin, was just a few hours away. The time ticked by slowly until finally I left my office and went two flights down to the first floor, registered at the reception desk, and settled myself into the patient waiting area. I resisted feeling part of it: magazines, newspapers, information pamphlets on cancer, and patients pretending to not notice each other.

I was called to a small conference room and shortly Agustin entered and extended his hand for a formal handshake.

"What do you know about your disease?" he asked as we both sat down.

"I know it is ovarian cancer. I know it has spread to my lymph nodes. I know I will need lots of chemotherapy."

"It's Stage IV ovarian cancer specifically primary peritoneal carcinoma," he said.

I shut my eyes and let this sink in. I heard myself exhale. Maybe my closed eyes were an attempt to shut this out, saying to myself that I would not let this in and hoping when I opened my eyes it would all be a bad dream, a nightmare. But it wasn't.

Somehow saying Stage IV seemed so much worse than saying it had spread. While I knew it was true, Agustin was the first to say it out loud to me. I had convinced myself that because I did not have a large mass in my abdomen that it was not so bad. Even for me, being knowledgeable about cancer, I was denying. I knew it was a form of self-protection that helped me to continue through the previous days to this appointment, sitting in that chair and hearing the dreaded "Stage IV." Of course, I had been fooling myself, I knew it had to be Stage IV. I had cancer everywhere, above and below the diaphragm, left and right side, all four quadrants; it was everywhere. When I opened my eyes, I realized I had to know the whole truth.

"Is it also in my lungs?"

"No."

"Is it in my brain?"

"No."

"Is it in my liver?"

"No."

"We don't see it any of those places," he said.

Even in the throes of horrible news, at least there was a bit of good news, a way to say it could be worse, and a perspective to maintain hope. There were parts of my body what were still healthy. Maybe I could build on that.

But still, I waited to hear what Agustin would say next. Would he say, "sorry we probably can't do anything but keep you comfortable and control your pain?" Would he say, "we can treat this but it is too far advanced and it probably won't do much good?" I really did not know what to expect him to say next.

Instead of pessimism and guarded stilted warnings, he seemed optimistic. He said there were good treatments. "Women survive this, not just rarely but every day." And then he talked about Lance Armstrong who had testicular cancer and it was in his brain and lungs but he went on to win the Tour de France after cancer. In retrospect, even though Armstrong was shown years later to have taken performance enhancing drugs, still he overcame cancer and regained his fitness and his example was important that day and it stays with me to this day. It did not seem that Agustin was simply giving me false hope because the alternative was too difficult to say. It seemed that he really believed that I could survive this even if he didn't think I would become a competitive cyclist.

That brief conversation sustained me through many difficult days. When I sat alone and said to myself "just thirty percent survive five years" I then said to myself "but Agustin thinks I could be in that thirty percent or 20%, or whatever smaller number it was for Stage IV. The fact is that I never asked Agustin my prognosis. I never said, "What are my chances of surviving?" I never said "How long do I have?" Because I knew, and he knew, that in the individual case, nobody knows. I was working to maintain hope. Agustin was optimistic, and so I accepted that, and tried to just get on with it. If I learned otherwise during treatment, maybe this attitude would have changed, but it seemed this was the best way to approach treatment at the outset. At least, this is how I wanted to start this unknown and uncertain dive into treatment. And not only did I want to believe I would survive; I began to believe there was a very good chance I would survive.

Quickly we moved on to talking about the treatment. The standard treatment is carboplatin and Taxol, two cytotoxic chemotherapy drugs every three weeks for six cycles. But Agustin wanted to be more aggressive. He wanted to give the Taxol every week for 18 weeks and he wanted to add another new drug, bevacizumab (Avastin) as well. This was a new antiangiogenesis drug. It worked by preventing the tumor from establishing its own blood supply. But he warned me that the FDA had not approved bevacizumab for gynecologic cancers, so the insurance company might not pay for it. (In fact, it was not approved until 2014). Nonetheless the studies to support it were in progress and Agustin expected that the first results would be coming out soon. He thought it would cost about $70,000 dollars if the insurance company denied payment and if I had to pay for it.

Still, I wanted a second opinion at another cancer center. Armed with my pathology reports, pathology slides, and CDs with pictures of my scans, I met with another expert in ovarian cancer. The slides were reviewed by another pathologist and confirmed. I was offered the standard treatment by the consulting physician. I decided to go with Agustin's more aggressive regimen. My reasoning came from a lecture I heard a long time ago given by a head and neck surgeon. His approach was "aggressive early and conservative late." This simply meant that he would do a big extensive surgery when he felt it was early enough to have a meaningful impact on survival, but he would be conservative later in the course of an illness and avoid major surgery when there was little chance of substantially affecting the outcome. With cancer, it is always beneficial to get a second opinion with regard to the diagnosis and the treatment and I felt more certain having done that.

Seeking out care for me was easy but I recognize that it is not easy for everyone. It is important for any patient to seek out the best care and to not settle for whatever doctor or hospital is close to home, or for a familiar hospital where other problems had been treated, or where a friend is on staff. Seeking expert care is critical and needs to be made during the height of anxiety. Some cancers, like ovarian, are rare or complex and there are physicians and medical teams that specialize in treating these cancers and it makes a big difference in providing state-of-the-art care.

This was my first treatment and I wanted to be aggressive. "Bring it on," I thought. "I can tolerate being miserable for 18 weeks. I am going to give this my best shot." No guarantees either way. Whatever extra edge the bevacizumab would give me, Jim and I were willing to pay for. Yes, it would make me angry if the insurance did not pay for my treatment. But why had I saved for retirement if I was not going to survive to see it? I had those savings and many people don't. Cost would be a barrier to optimal care for poor women. Would they die because they couldn't commit to this expense? Should they go bankrupt in order to try? It was not clear if this drug would actually help me or if it was just an expensive lure that I was trying to catch. But I had the money. I could take a chance. Spend it now, I decided.

*

National data report the life expectancy at 5 years is only 19% for Stage IV ovarian cancer. But since I was in otherwise good health, I decided it was really 30% for me. And because I had access to the best medical care, and worked at the hospital where I would be treated, and personally knew my oncologist, nurses, pathologist, phlebotomist and surgeon, I decided it was really more like 35%. And I thought, "why shouldn't I be in that 35%," even if it's really 25%, or even 19%. But it was all just numbers. Nobody could predict exactly what would happen to me. If I survived it would be 100%. If I died, it would be 0%. That was the reality.

But with cancer there are big unknowns. Will the chemo work? Will it help me or will it kill me? Will my body tolerate the chemo or will the toxicity be so bad that they can't treat me? Will the cancer be resistant to the chemo or will those cancer cells die? Will I go into remission? Will the cancer recur? This last question is the most frightening about ovarian cancer. It often comes back. For me, with Stage IV, the chance of surviving five years without ever having a recurrence was under 10%, bad odds but not zero.

These questions filled my head in the fall of 2010. I felt I had little control over how well the chemo would work. I could not will my healthy cells to survive despite the use of those toxic drugs. I could not will the cancer cells to die when exposed to the same drugs. I was rooting for the healthy cells in my body to thrive while wishing death on the cancerous others.

Cancer was my enemy. Chemo, I decided, would be my friend. I thought of chemo as my friend PITA — Pain in The Ass chemo. The challenge would be to get through 18 weeks with my aggressive chemo friend PITA. PITA might make me sick at times and we might not always be on the best terms, but I was hoping that friend would grant me years of life. What would that chemo be like I wondered? For the next 18 weeks, my Tuesdays would belong to chemo but the other six days of the week were mine. I was determined to try to live my life as normally as I could despite the cancer.

Chapter 4: Stage IV

For thirty years before I was diagnosed, I conducted studies to understand how people deal with the diagnosis and treatments for cancer or for AIDS. I studied how people complied with the medications, dealt with the side effects, disclosed to family and friends, continued working, exercising and managing their fears. I developed programs to help people with these challenges. I studied how to manage familial risk for cancer. I developed national programs to reduce high-risk sexual behavior and non-disclosure on the part of HIV positive patients and I had worked with the CDC to disseminate these HIV prevention programs.

So, it was not surprising that when the time came for me to deal with my own cancer diagnosis, I had already thought through many of the challenges I would face. In many ways I was a very prepared patient. I knew what I needed to do. I found that I was almost observing myself from an objective distance to see whether I could do what I knew I was required to do. And in some ways, I felt I wanted to be and needed to be the model patient. So, while my background prepared me more than most, it was also a test to see if I could practice what I had learned. But thinking about and studying cancer is very different from experiencing it.

The most common question that people ask when they learn that someone has cancer is, "What stage is it?" The answer of "Stage IV" is almost synonymous with death. Staging is a tricky business – there are people who live and people who die at every stage, so stage gives a probability answer about prognosis but the answer is incomplete, because it can never provide a particular patient with his or her certain prognosis. We are people after all and not probability numbers.

Stage IV was frightening enough to me, let alone having to say it over and over again, "It is Stage IV" as I watched the response. So, when people asked, I did not answer that question directly. Instead, I said, "I have cancer on my peritoneum and in my lymph nodes, but it is not in my liver, lungs, brain, or bones." For most people, this more detailed and specific information sounded confusing and perhaps it lessened their concern. Some even said "that's good." To be honest, that was very good. I was thankful for those still safe parts of my body, but I was also intentionally obfuscating.

Most people have a difficult time talking to someone who is newly diagnosed with cancer. With all good intentions, they are nervous and anxious and they don't know what to say. They want to express concern and ask how things are going but behind that there is often the dark lurking question, "How long have you got?"

But in everyday interactions, until the hair went, nobody would have suspected that I had Stage IV cancer. At times I wanted to tell people and at times I wanted to hide it. And then I got irritated with those who couldn't see what I was going through. When I went to the grocery store, the checker was rude and distracted. She wouldn't make eye contact. She was brusque and unpleasant. She spoke in one syllable dialog. "Fifty-one dollars, 34 cents." "Bags?" "Card." She should have been nicer to me I thought. "I have cancer and I am barely functioning to come to this store and buy groceries. Don't you realize you are making my already miserable day worse? Can't you tell?" But of course, she could not tell and maybe it would have made a difference but maybe not. I didn't say thank you when I left.

Upon reflection, this experience was a lesson to me. You can't tell the difficulties that others are experiencing. Maybe her day was worse than mine. But I doubt it. Still, I cannot tell the challenges others are going through nor can they tell mine. So be kind.

Because I worked in a cancer center, my colleagues knew what Stage IV ovarian cancer meant. I did not need to explain it. Recurrences are common with ovarian cancer and entail more treatment and possibly remission, but then another recurrence and more treatment and scans and more chemo and possibly more surgery. But all of the efforts could end up with diminishing returns and no good options left.

But maybe all of these assumptions about Stage IV and what it would lead to for me were wrong. Maybe this did not have to be the case. Maybe in my case it would be chemo and surgery and then walking and working and remission and no recurrence and life again. Others had recovered and never recurred, the "one and done" survivors. And I was wondering how to get myself among those exceptional responders. But still, it was Stage IV and there was no denying it was serious. I spent hours trying to figure out how to survive and I knew that whatever I did there was much I would not be able to control. My mind went back and forth between hope and fear.

Chapter 5: Centering Myself — Gratitude, Integrity and Determination

Cancer is living with uncertainty but so is life, it's just that cancer makes the uncertainty a daily thought. Nobody knows the number of our days, not even with Stage IV disease. Nobody knows.

And then the question changed for me, or more accurately the questions expanded. What kind of person did I want to be as I worked through this? How did I want to go through treatment? What kind of wife, mother, and grandmother, what kind of friend, colleague, and mentor did I want to be going through cancer? And here my life work in a cancer center felt like it both informed me and gave me a path that I needed to stay on.

There were decisions to be made. I could decide how I would interact with others, how I would answer their questions, what I would do with my time, who I would surround myself with, how I would work, how I would parent and how I would care for myself. As long as I was alive, I was not just a body to be worked on — I had decisions to make and I was still responsible for my behavior, thoughts and emotions. Cancer did not absolve me of any of this. I needed to figure out how to live with this in the present moment and how to believe in and construct my future. And if the treatment did not work, I would need to decide how I would die. But that decision was in the future. Right then, it was about how I would meet these challenges head on.

My cancer diagnosis and treatment created a fissure in my life, a disruption, an assault that had to be lived through. Millions of people had experienced what I was experiencing and millions had survived the grueling treatment necessary. But I needed to figure it out for myself. How would I live with the fear and panic? How would I not become a burden? How would I still feel joy? How would I experience life and not let the shadow engulf me?

Jean LeCerf Richardson

There is a poem titled *The Summer Day* by Mary Oliver. Like many of her poems, it seems to start with an observance of nature and then asks or offers some thoughtful reflection on how to be fully human in this life. In this poem, she asks what the reader plans to do with her one life, her one wild and precious life. And with cancer, the length of my life was in question and how to spend my time was looming over me.

The question Mary Oliver raised, alone and out of context seemed an exhortation to do more, achieve more, shake things up, be outstanding. In the past, I felt these words directed me to travel more, to take chances, and to take on challenges outside of my comfortable academic life. Maybe they said to dance all night or maybe to follow Cheryl Strayed as she told her story in *Wild*, and walk the Pacific Crest Trail, alone and unprepared, to be wild.

But in her preceding lines, Mary Oliver wrote about a walk through a meadow and the small observance of a grasshopper eating and washing itself. Was this common and small joy enough to answer her question? Was the answer to wander, to idle, to observe nature, and write a poem about a grasshopper? Did this measure up and was this a satisfying answer to her question?

But the second to the last line is rarely quoted. She asks if everything dies and all too soon. I knew the answer to that one. "Yes, no question — life is short." Life is too short for us and for the grasshopper she was looking at. And if everything dies too soon, what do you do with the life you have — your precious life? How do you choose to live?

The two lines together were the real message for me. The words came into sharper focus when death hovered near, when threat surrounded, when fear grew, when cancer came. How would I live my only life, the life uniquely my own, now that I had cancer and now that I fully realized how short my life might be? Was mine a life in retreat or could I choose?

While fear, panic and anxiety seemed natural, I knew that if I allowed these feelings to dominate my life, I would be miserable and likely make those I love miserable as well. In the end it would not help. I did not want to be *that* person living through cancer. I did not want to lose myself or to change into a whimpering, angry, broken, or fatalistic person. I wanted to get through this in a way that was consistent with who I wanted to be. I believed if I could do that, then I would improve my chances of surviving.

I had studied issues related to adapting to chronic serious diseases. I knew that studies had shown healthy people who were depressed had a shorter survival time. This was also true for people with cancer, AIDS or heart disease. Whether it is because depression interferes with other life supporting activities such as compliance with treatment or exercise, or because it works through poorly understood biological, possibly immunologic, pathways. Over and over again the negative burden of depression has been confirmed in study after study and this was not who I wanted to be. This does not mean taking on the mantle of toxic positivity, but it does mean avoiding depression.

I remembered my mother as she lived with cancer. She maintained her interest in life and in friends and family throughout; she did what she could when she could. Even while her world narrowed, she never did. Her struggle prepared me for my own struggle.

I wanted to show my children how to live through cancer because some day they might need to do the same. The thought that years in the future my children might need a role model even if I was no longer alive, and that in my attention to the disease and my response to it, I would help them in whatever they might face that was unwanted and frightening. This gave me strength.

It is generational strength. In a family you learn from each other and when one falls the others become the support to stand up again. Usually, it is the parent lifting the child, but with age, it can become the child lifting the parent. Families build resilience in each other, even over generations. My mother had taught me how to face cancer and I would need to teach my children; all the time hoping they would never face this.

Feelings are not inevitable, and neither is behavior. Without thought, feelings could be like dry leaves in the wind – blown and piled carelessly. I had decisions to make about what values I would bring to this experience. I needed to articulate words to myself that would help me lean on my values, that I could rely on and cling to. These words would keep me from being driven down by the bad chemo effects, from unwelcome comments, from seeing myself in a chemo chair every week, and from uncertainty. These would be my strength. Little by little I began to find the words and the intention of how I wanted to see myself, who I wanted to be and what I would do with my precious life.

What did it mean to ground or center myself in a word? In the past, grounding myself in the word "kind," forced me to check myself in any number of circumstances and ask myself if I was being kind. Through *intention* to live the word "kind" I became kinder. But "kind" was not the right word for cancer. "Kind" led me out into the world and cancer felt more like an internal battle. The words I needed would tell me how I wanted to live. As I reflected on this while I was buffeted by the worries and the uncertainty of cancer, I began to ground myself in the words *gratitude, integrity,* and *determination.*

Where did *gratitude* come from after the cancer diagnosis? It was not gratitude for the cancer but it was gratitude for much else. I was 61 years old when I was diagnosed. I was grateful for 61 healthy years. I was not a child, nor was the cancer affecting my children or my grandchildren. Every parent I know who has had a child with cancer would trade places with that child. I was grateful it was me, and not them.

I was grateful for a long marriage to a good man. Jim and I had been married for 41 years. We married when I was 20 and he was 22, which now seems outrageously young to get married. In spite of that, we supported each other through advanced degrees. We had our first child Katherine when I was 25 and our son David followed three years later. We are perhaps a nerdy pair, we both read broadly, he seeks out books on science, astronomy, history, theology and philosophy while I read about biology and nature as well as biographies and novels. Jim is a master woodworker and a gift of his woodwork for weddings, graduations, and anniversaries is a lucky treasure. We have hiked and camped for our entire marriage. He shies away from medical settings and I am comfortable there. As with any long marriage, we have supported each other through good times and bad, and I realized we were going to go into the part about "in sickness and in health" and while I was more comfortable in the supportive role in medical settings, he was going to need to support me during this treatment. Jim's father had died when he was just 12 and his mother died in 2009, almost exactly one year before I was diagnosed. And we did not know it at the time, but his brother would die in 2011 after many years of poor health, and before I finished chemo. Through those three years of grief and worry, I knew I could count on Jim to help me get through cancer.

Katherine was happily married to her husband Mike and David to his wife Ali. And they each had healthy and happy children of their own. Surprisingly, they each had baby boys in 2007 and they each had their second sons in 2009. Our four little grandsons were so young that Jim and I were new at the joy of being grandparents. I was afraid that the only thing they might ever remember about me, if they remembered me at all, was that

I was sick and that thought hung on me like dead leaves. I felt proud of the children Jim and I had raised and for that I felt grateful.

I had many blessings in my life including my parents who represented everything that is implied in the term "the greatest generation" honest, hardworking, modest, and thoughtful – survivors of the Great Depression and my Dad, a veteran of World War II.

I was grateful for my meaningful and fulfilling career. I was grateful for friends and family who walked with me through life's challenges and joys. I was grateful to have access to my medical team, and I was grateful for the strong chemotherapy. While cancer does not discriminate, access to medical care does, and my access made survival possible for me. Gratitude was a reminder from childhood, "count your blessings not your complaints."

With the word *integrity* I thought about honesty, but more. I thought about wholeness and adherence to values of justice. At a deeper sense integrity meant keeping myself intact. If a building or a wall fell down in a storm or in an earthquake, I might question how well it was built. Was it fractured? Did it have steel reinforcements? Were cheap materials used? Did it have integrity? For me, "integrity" meant strength and wholeness. It meant attention to structure and intent to live in a way to resist damage, it meant keeping my sense of self throughout.

To me, *determination* was not just a word about mental attitude – it also meant doing what I needed to do. It meant pushing for a quick diagnosis and start of therapy, getting a second opinion, continuing to exercise, eating as I was able to, showing up for all of the chemo and doctors visits, living with the discomfort of chemo and surgery, continuing to work, trying to keep my life as normal as possible, and pushing back on depression and mental fatigue.

Cancer lurked in the corners of my mind, and I needed to firmly tell that dark shadow to leave me alone so I could live my life as well as I could, with purpose even during cancer. What will I do with my life when death might be sooner than I expected, when I could see how short life now seemed? What will I do with my one life which was precious to me but certainly did not feel wild as I looked forward? What will I do when the treatment itself would keep me from truly enjoying my life and then might not work at all? Cancer could bring me to my knees, but I was not going to be buffeted day to day, I was not going to be helpless in this storm. Mary Oliver's question in her poem was my question, and it needed to be thought about and answered. What would I do with my wild and precious life? My three words strengthened my intention to find a way to tolerate the treatment and to live with purpose. But even with all intention to feel otherwise, I struggled and I suspect that most people with cancer endure a similar struggle. How to contemplate death and still live a life of purpose.

PART II: CHEMOTHERAPY — MY PITA (PAIN IN THE ASS) FRIEND

Chapter 6: The Kardashians and Other Amusements During Chemo

When I think about being on chemo and try to explain what it felt like, maybe the most honest thing I could say is it drove me, a scientist, to watch the Kardashians.

"Have you ever watched the Kardashians?"

"What?" my friends Susan, Sue, and Yvonne asked together wondering what the heck I was talking about. Jim started to laugh.

I was lying in the chemo infusion bed getting hooked up for my weekly doses of chemo surrounded by four people in a tight circle inside the curtained enclosure.

"You know, those women with that show that is all about themselves and their stuff and their social life. You know, the Kardashians. I watched it the other day."

"Oh my God," said Yvonne, "what's happening to you? That's crazy," and she started laughing.

True enough. I couldn't argue the point.

And then my nurse Imelda rushed in and checked my infusion pump, "I love their clothes," she said catching the end of the conversation. And then she was off to the next bed leaving us startled and then laughing out loud.

"It's so ridiculous," I said leaving them to wonder if I was talking about the show or about me watching it.

I learned as I went through chemotherapy to expect some down days when I had no energy, could not read, and could not eat. I watched daytime TV to take my mind off of myself and my own unanswerable questions. I would slowly pet Jackson, my black Lab, while learning to cook beef bourguignon when I could only drink milkshakes. I watched home repair and decorating shows where women like me were knocking out walls with sledge hammers so they could have an "open concept" home and painting their rooms various shades of grey or taupe. "What have they got against color?" I wondered. I watched shows where gay men helped girls pick out their wedding dresses. I watched Ellen DeGeneres dance when I was having trouble walking on my neuropathy feet. And I watched President Obama's determination to get a health care plan enacted so that millions of Americans would get health care. All the while, I could barely figure out the statements I was getting weekly from hospitals and insurance companies. And I wondered how cancer patients who did not have health insurance could possibly survive a cancer diagnosis; and the obvious answer was that they were far less likely to survive. And I also realized I was now among those with a preexisting condition, and from then on, insurance companies would prefer to get rid me and my profit draining problems. And so, I cheered Obama on.

And one afternoon out of curiosity, I even watched the Kardashians. But my chemo brain could not figure out the plot or the point. What was that show about anyway? Was it my chemo brain or was the show really a parade of pointless display?

"Not much on daytime TV."

"She is watching "Hallmark Hall of Fame" movies," Jim groaned.

And it was true. Everything always worked out. Those sticky, sweet, formulaic movies where the girl and guy at first do not get along and one or the other was already hooked up with the completely wrong partner. Then through a series of mishaps, they discover that they are in love, the wrong partner gets dumped, and they finally get together. They are a hundred versions of *Pride and Prejudice.* Yes, these didn't demand much thought. And they always worked out just as I knew they should and would. It was predictable and when nothing else felt predictable, it was comforting to know that at least in Hallmark-land, I could predict the outcome with certainty and I'd always be right.

I learned that whatever I did to get through chemo was a good thing and not to be judged by anyone and especially by myself. The point was to get through it no matter how low my TV viewing might go.

What was chemo like? I have my stories and I have spent enough time with other patients to know a few things.

First, chemo is not the same for everyone. Bodies react differently to the cancer and to the treatment.

Second, chemo may cause reactions that are unexpected and some can be controlled and some cannot.

Third, chemo is a wait-and-see game to even know if it's working.

And finally, chemo is essential for some types of cancer, and mine was one of those. I had to depend on it to eradicate this cancer.

I can describe my experience with chemo – but it is only that – my experience, and I suspect that others may experience some of the same reactions as well as different ones. But I do believe that sharing information about chemo is helpful. And what was also helpful was that I knew I would get through it just as hundreds of thousands of others had done.

But I am getting ahead of myself. Chemo is a step-by-step process so it may be best to describe the steps from the beginning to the end and not start with watching all of the pointless TV that chemo drove me to on days when I just needed to stay still and let my body heal.

Chapter 7: Who Do I Tell? How Do I Tell?

At the end of August, Jim and I had plans to go to Gladstone's, a famous seafood restaurant in Malibu, for lunch with Katherine and her husband Mike to celebrate his birthday. In the week before that birthday celebration, I was going through all of the confusing tests to find out what was wrong with me but I had not yet received the confirmed diagnosis. I needed to tell them in person about what was happening but was stewing about ruining the day. We drove to their house so we could carpool to the beach in their minivan. I wish there was an easy way to break such bad news but if there is, I don't have that skill. As the two little boys, Connor three years old and Ryan just one, were busy playing on the grass, we simply blurted it out. The children were too young to understand the words or importance of what we were talking about or even to interrupt their play to listen. As I looked at the boys, I felt the fear that I would not be part of their lives for very long.

"I have cancer," I said.

I could see the shock on Katherine and Mikes' faces as they asked questions and we talked quietly about what this meant. We explained the diagnostic tests that I was going through and the uncertainty that was finally coming to a diagnosis, and the expectation that chemo would start soon.

"I am feeling fine. They are not certain but they think it is in my ovaries. I will be fine. I have good doctors. I will need chemotherapy, I know that."

"Maybe we shouldn't go out," they said.

"Why not? I'm looking forward to the beach and to lunch, it will be good for us" I said. "I really want to go."

I did feel fine physically although I could not say the same for my thoughts. We had all looked forward to good food, sitting on the sand and wading in the water. It would be good for Jim and me to get out and have a day of enjoyment before the final tests and the start of chemo. Perhaps that might lift the obsessive thinking about my cancer and what would happen next.

Normally at Gladstone's, I would eat too much. But, on this day I could barely eat. We walked on the beach but my mind was spinning. As I looked at my little grandsons playing on the sand, I wished for them to have many carefree days, to be healthy, to play without worry of the future. That worry was meant for adults not for children.

My son David lives in Rhode Island. I knew he was going on a research vessel for ocean sampling but I could not remember exactly what day he was leaving. When I called, his wife Ali said he was on the ship but it had pulled into port for bad weather conditions and to call him on his cell phone. When I reached him, he sounded shaken by the news. Perhaps I should have waited to tell him. I reassured him that I was going to start treatment soon. But he needed to keep his focus on what he was doing. "Keep your wits about you on the ship," I said, "you need to stay safe." A research vessel in the ocean is not a place to get careless or distracted.

David and Ali also had two little boys, Thomas and Trevor. I felt all of the hopes I had for being a grandparent to my four little grandsons beginning to evaporate; as the dreams of good times ahead began to narrow, I could feel the tears welling.

Then I called my brother. Once I told him I had cancer I started crying and I could not speak. I needed to hand the phone to Jim. Perhaps it was because we had both watched our mother die from cancer and those memories came flooding back. Or perhaps it reminded me that the comfort my mother would have provided if she were alive, would never be available to me. Or maybe it was just because we have a sibling bond of trust. He flew to California right away and we spent a few days together before the chemo started. I had not really come to grips with the diagnosis yet.

*

Working on the third floor of the cancer center while receiving infusions in the first-floor day hospital, made privacy impossible. There is no way to be treated in the same building where my office was upstairs and expect to keep my condition private - and for what purpose? I knew I needed to figure out the whole disclosure issue; how was I going to tell people and how was I going to maintain some privacy? I had studied disclosure among young men who had been diagnosed with AIDS and it was clear that some of those who disclosed suffered some negative responses from family, employers or friends. On the other hand, those who disclosed were more likely to find people who would support them through their illness than those who kept it secret. They did not suffer alone.

I knew there were people I wanted to tell personally to get ahead of the news as it spread through casual conversation.

I called Sue who had worked with me since 1997. "Can you get away for a short walk," I asked her, "there is something important I need to talk with you about." We walked around the East Los Angeles streets surrounding the USC health campus. As I told her, I saw the tears in her eyes.

"I think I am going to be alright," I said, "but you are going to hear bad things about this diagnosis so just don't believe them, I have a lot going for me."

"I will be there," she said. Good to her word she came to sit with me for a while during every one of my chemo infusions for 18 weeks.

One by one, I began to tell my colleagues. It took so much emotional energy to do this, that I could only manage a few a day.

When the diagnosis was determined and I was ready to begin chemo, I told my Institute director, Mary Ann, that I would write a note and asked her to read it to my colleagues at a division faculty meeting. I wanted to control the message and I did not want people learning, perhaps erroneous information, through gossip. I did not want any of them to learn from someone else and then wonder why they were the last to know and not the first.

Dear Friends

The last few weeks have been difficult to comprehend. I have been diagnosed with primary peritoneal cancer. Simply put, this is a rare form of ovarian cancer that is silent in terms of symptoms and is not detected by any of our routine cancer screening methods. This is a serious disease but there are now new effective chemotherapeutic treatments for it and I have good reason to be optimistic. I will be having chemotherapy for the next 5 months. I have had excellent care through the process of reaching a diagnosis with many of the doctors doing the CT scans, biopsies and pathology as well as the oncologists being personal friends. For this I am grateful.

I have studied issues of cancer and AIDS screening, early detection and patient issues in treatment for my entire career. There is no question that this will change my insight into all of these issues and I will learn from it.

I am otherwise healthy. Three weeks ago, I was hiking, whitewater rafting and kayaking in Yellowstone. On the weekend I am riding my horse and I am walking every day. I tell you this so that you know that I am feeling well and I am learning to deal with this disease and am ready to get started on treatment on Wednesday.

I intend to continue working through the treatment and the physicians have encouraged me to do that. I am reachable by email even if I am not in the office. I asked Mary Ann to keep this confidential until the diagnosis was reached which it now is. I have asked her to tell you as a group. I would appreciate your prayers.

With Love to you all
Jean

But this note was not completely true. There were not new and effective chemotherapy treatments. Unfortunately, the survival rates had not been improving. I would be given the standard chemotherapy of carboplatin and Taxol that had been around for over 20 years and was the core of my treatment although weekly dosing with Taxol and adding bevacizumab was a new approach. I did not tell them it was Stage IV and that it had spread throughout my body. However, the oncologist and surgeon did give me hope and encouraged optimism — even as the statistics on the disease were pessimistic.

Some days I found myself comforting colleagues and telling them that I expected to survive and be well again. One of my former doctoral students had lost her mother to this disease and now she was afraid she might lose her mentor to the very same disease. With my diagnosis, the sad memories came rushing back and she could not hide the tears. She had been the one to translate from the physician to her Spanish-speaking mother throughout her mother's care. I knew she was crying for her mother who had died young, as well as for me.

There were days as I walked around the cancer center that I felt some colleagues saw me as "dead woman walking." I may have looked the same but I was different and those who knew about the cancer could see it. And among those who could see it were some who already anticipated my death. They knew the data but they did not know what would happen to me, nobody could know that until the treatment was complete and several years had passed. I learned that people have differing abilities to be supportive or obtuse under these circumstances. Even though they meant no harm, years later, I still remember statements that felt unkind at the time and those that felt supportive. In times of crisis and stress, some things are forgotten but not unkind or insensitive words and not kindness or supportive words either.

I remember:

a colleague who ducked into an office when she saw me coming down the hall and was clearly avoiding me.

three colleagues and my husband who were there for every chemo infusion.

a colleague who wasn't feeling well and responded to my news with "At least you know what is wrong with you."

a colleague who hugged me and said, "I've got your back – I'm here."

a friend who visited and ended up talking about his own long-term health challenges, who even after I had helped him for years and given blood for his surgeries, I realized he couldn't put himself aside and express interest or concern for me.

a friend who said "NO, you are going to be fine – just fine."

a friend who said, "In five years we will still be walking together."

When I said to another colleague that I planned to still be alive in five years, he asked, "How do you know that?"

But maybe he was right. Nobody knew for sure.

And then there were those who kept their distance, no phone calls, no emails, and no visits. At some level these were the most disappointing.

I asked myself, "What is it about cancer that makes people ask unanswerable questions? How is it that anyone dare ask me, "How long did they say you have?"

And then there are those who just blurt out their straight question. "Are you going to die?" leaving both of us speechless as the question hangs in the air between us. And the people who ask, are people who do care about me but simply don't know what to say or maybe they think being harshly honest is a good interaction. Yes of course, people wonder if that is the case. All the while I felt like I had been hit in the head with a brick as I control myself and respond, "No, I am starting treatment, I don't know what will happen, but my doctors are optimistic and so am I."

It is a surprising thing that happens when you are diagnosed with cancer. People want to tell you stories of other people they know who died of cancer and of how hard it was on everyone around them. One colleague told me of a friend who was a seven-year survivor. My comfort was quickly dashed when he then said it had been a miserable seven years. Not helpful. Really why did I need to hear about the best friend of my accountant's wife who died of ovarian cancer? Why did I need to hear about the sister-in-law of a colleague who had ovarian cancer? Bottom line is, unless they were alive and well and riding a bike to work every day, I didn't really need to hear it.

While everyone who I was close to knew about the diagnosis and all of my colleagues knew, I waffled between telling and not telling those who were more casual contacts. Because cancer was always on my mind, it was sometimes hard for me to keep it out of conversations. On the other hand, did I expect anything other than "I am sorry to hear this" from casual friendships?

It was critically important for me to be supported during my cancer treatment by those who were close friends and family. It was profoundly disappointing when those I expected to be supportive seemed to drift away. The issue here is expectations and reciprocation. If I expected someone to be supportive and they were not, it was destructive. If I had supported them in prior difficulties of any sort and they did not reciprocate, it was destructive. And so, some relationships cooled and some ended. While other relationships were strengthened and endured. As I have talked with many women with cancer, it has become clear to me that this is true for almost all of them; some friends and family step up and some don't, some help and some disappear, some approach and some run away. You can't make someone who is not helpful into the person you want them to be at that time. You don't have the power to fix or even understand them. As you recognize who they are, you let go of who you want them to be. Holding on, expecting more, getting angry — none of it changes them it only mires you with a disease and with anger, a combination that does not promote healing. And then you find the helpers and those relationships deepen and get you through. And that is the blessing. Those people are the ones you will keep.

People often wonder what to do for a friend with cancer. The obvious answer is "do something." But here are some thoughts. Calls and emails are appreciated. One of my friends with cancer got so many calls that his children got annoyed. But he simply told them "How would it feel if no one called?" So, call and be willing to keep it short. Besides that, friends gave me books, food, hats and scarves, green tea, turmeric tea, plants, heating pads, lotions, potions, totems (ethnic totems for good health) and shawls. People also came and watched TV with me, took me to breakfast or lunch, packed up my office when our department was relocated, called me during sports events that we "watched" together, walked with me after surgery, picked me up to go to the Arboretum, and sat with me while I was waiting in clinic and while I had chemo. Cancer therapy often feels like a very long lonely rainy day and human kindness makes it bearable.

Chapter 8: Trepidations, Prayers and Omens

Monday was Labor Day. Tuesday, I went in for blood tests, a final CT scan, and a PET scan, in preparation for starting chemo on Wednesday.

The nurse who did the scans had short spiked hair. Her face was angular and bright. She told me that she was a breast cancer survivor and she went through all of these scans as well. She told me that some days she would just sit in a chair hugging herself, and telling herself, "I will be well." She lost her hair and when she went to yoga with a scarf on her head it kept falling off until the teacher told her to forget that scarf. When she went to yoga class the next time, her bald head led the way in downward dog and she felt cared for and not embarrassed. Even though this was just a little story, her words helped me.

Again, I was shoved in and out of the scanner, holding my breath and staying still, with my arms above my head. Though it might seem easy, the scan was frightening, it was hard for me to keep calm and not move inside the machine as it took cross sectional pictures of my body for the CT scan. The PET scan used radioactive tagged sugar, which accumulated in any places the cancer had spread. On the PET scan image, all of those places would light up.

I chanted to myself through the CT and PET scans and recited the 23rd psalm over and over again. It is the psalm of comfort when facing the fear of death. And it is the only psalm I can remember.

Yea though I walk through the valley of the shadow of death
I will fear no evil for though art with me
Thy rod and thy staff they comfort me

I learned this psalm as a child. When I say it, I feel a connection with the prayers of others over the centuries. Reciting it to myself over and over again focused and calmed my nervous brain and it kept me still.

As expected, the CT and PET scans showed abnormal lymph nodes throughout my body. The PET scan was lit up like a poorly decorated Christmas tree, marking the cancer in all those lymph nodes just as Mabel had said.

*

It was September 8, 2010. Rosh Hashanah would begin at sundown. It was raining in Los Angeles. It was my first day of chemotherapy. I wondered whether the rain and Rosh Hashanah were fraught with meaning that I could not discern but would foreshadow what was going to happen with the cancer and with my life.

Rain in September in Los Angeles is rare, and because the summers are hot and dry and water itself is precious, it could only mean new life. Life to the brown and thirsty grass, the drooping flowers, and my redwood tree that should have been growing along a misty coast but instead was sixty feet tall and 12 feet around in my front yard. That redwood and two across the street were struggling but surviving with a little help from deep watering through those dry months of summer. Was this tree a totem for me? Get some help, get deep water, survive another year. Had I been on the east coast where I grew up, I would have seen it as just another rainy day, but in California, rain was a reason for joy. Be grateful for the rain. A good omen.

When did I start looking for omens? I was a scientist. I didn't look for omens; I looked for data. "I want the information and conclusions and I want to know the facts that support those conclusions." But all I really knew was that I had Stage IV disease, it was everywhere, it was moving fast and mutating as it went. The outlook was not good. And, I didn't want to dwell on those facts and perhaps that was why I was looking for omens and signs instead. We find omens when we need them and I needed them.

As I look back on my day planner from 2010, I see it in big letters on September 8. "CHEMO STARTS" and in the preprinted notation "Rosh Hashanah begins at sundown." I remember that I looked it up. Rosh Hashanah, I knew was the Jewish New Year, the Day of Judgment and 10 days later was Yom Kippur, the Day of Atonement.

Rosh Hashanah is a time of prayer but also a day of judgment. It begins the ten-day period of atonement for individual and communal sins over the previous year ending in Yom Kippur, the Day of Atonement. Wishes and greetings are exchanged for a good year. But, one of the prayers says "all inhabitants of the world pass before G-d like a flock of sheep, and it is decreed in the heavenly court who shall live, and who shall die… who shall be impoverished and who shall be enriched; who shall fall and who shall rise." On that day, G-d closes the books and our fate is inscribed for the coming year and names of the righteous are written and sealed in the Book of Life. Two of my Jewish friends had gone to temple and prayed for me on that holy day and that felt like a blessing.

I wondered if the days of judgment were a good omen or a bad omen and if, at the judgment, I would fall or rise, and if I would live or die. It was all too easy to conflate the judgmental lore of a cancer diagnosis with the belief that God judges and after all, it was the judging season. Was this cancer a punishment for a real or imagined event, a behavior or a sin? Would my name be written in the Book of Life or would God give up on me? And did any of this make sense in my otherwise scientific mind. While I am no atheist, I cannot say I am a fervent and consistent believer either. Maybe cancer reaches into that part of the soul that speaks to God or maybe it is simply that throwing these prayers out into the universe, whether there is any spirit to hear them or not, is just the human response to fear and powerlessness.

Rain could signal the flood and Rosh Hashanah could signal judgment. But they both could signal new life and that is what I chose to believe. Omens and signs were about seeking magic, to put a shred of meaning to what I chose to believe amid confusion. Somehow for me the first day of chemo on Rosh Hashanah seemed more than magical, it seemed like a blessing. And rain, so unlikely the first week of September seemed like an omen, a gift. I decided these were good signs, signs of new life. I held onto them like being suspended on a spider thread. I held onto them like Adam touching God's finger on the Sistine ceiling. I held onto them while standing squarely next to my redwood tree and seeing the rain sustain its life.

Chapter 9: Cycle 1 (Weeks 1-3) — I Got This

As Jim and I drove to the hospital for my first day of chemo, all we could do was listen to NPR, or more truthfully, NPR was on the radio, which was good, since we could not carry on a conversation ourselves. Jim and I are quiet people, but on that day, we were quieter than usual, even for us. Somehow words were impossible to find, the unknown and uncertainty was so heavy for us that both small talk and meaningful talk were too much, and we both retreated into our own thoughts.

"I hope this goes well," I ventured.

"You will be fine," he said.

"I know," I said.

But the fact was that neither of us knew anything about "fine" right then. We could hear the uncertainty in each other's voices.

And the process began. Get in line at reception, check in and show my patient card. Go to the blood draw clinic and wait to be called. Show my patient card and get several tubes of blood drawn, hopefully by my favorite phlebotomist. Sit in the waiting room and wait to be called for my appointment to see Agustin. Get called into the exam room by Michelle.

Michelle, one of the nurses who I would get to know began the process of weighing and measuring. "How tall are you? Dr. Garcia said 'tall' but I think we need more accuracy than that to figure out the right dosage of the chemo."

I stretched to my full height. "Five foot eight exactly." "Good for me," I thought, "at least I haven't shrunk."

She asked how I had been feeling. I told her about my mild symptoms, that I hiked and rode horses with a bunch of teenagers, and at 61 years old and with no illnesses, I thought I was super woman and not aging. "And then this. It has been a shock," I said. And more than that it was a profound disappointment in my own body, I felt let down and the shock had not yet worn off.

"It always is, nobody sees it coming," she said, and I knew she had probably heard this hundreds of times.

"Have you noticed any other changes?" she asked.

"The CT scan showed I have an enlarged lymph node in my armpit that I never noticed. It's deep down near my ribs and it feels like a shooter marble, an inch across under my skin. When I push on it, it feels sore. The scan shows lots more, but this is the only one close enough to the surface to feel."

"Dr. Garcia will want to examine that," she said, "he will be in shortly."

I knew Agustin as a colleague but we had never worked together on a project and our interactions had been loose pleasantries. He is small and trim with dark, curly hair and always seemed to me to have a slightly bemused look about him. I thought he might have a quirky sense of humor. I didn't know how he would be as a personal physician. I was curious.

But it did feel awkward for me. I was a senior faculty member but at that moment I felt powerless, not like a senior respected anything. Agustin and I were on a first name basis and that helped to maintain some dignity that was quickly getting lost as I transitioned from a cancer researcher to a cancer patient. A patient. Who was the first person to call sick people patients? It is a silly play on words. I certainly didn't feel patient but I knew I would need to be just that. I knew I would need to be patient with uncertainty and with my own body. "Patience is a virtue," revolved in my brain. Who taught me that? I couldn't even remember.

When Agustin came into the exam room, I introduced Jim. He shook hands with both of us. This formality was repeated at every visit over our long time together. To me it indicated mutual respect and I liked it. We got off to a good start, particularly for Jim, who is uncomfortable in medical settings. Simply shaking hands with Agustin was an invitation to participate.

When Agustin palpated the enlarged node in my armpit, he asked, "How long has it been there?"

"I don't know," I replied, I had a breast exam a month ago and the doctor did not notice it. I never felt it either until after the CT scan showed it was there and then after I knew it was there, I was able to feel it."

Agustin closed his eyes mentally measuring the node with his fingers.

"What's the plan?" I asked, "I know I am in for a lot of chemo."

"A study in Japan showed better results with weekly chemo," he said. I want you to have three drugs: carboplatin, and bevacizumab every three weeks and Taxol every week. The Taxol is 50% of a normal dose but over three weeks you will be getting 150%. Bevacizumab is usually given if there is a recurrence but I want to give it all up front. I think together these will work better. There are several ongoing trials so we will know more soon." He was willing to try something new and I was all for it.

"Every week?" I asked.

"Yes," he said, "for 18 weeks. Week one will be all three drugs and then two weeks of Taxol only. That will be repeated for six cycles."

"Throw it at me," I thought, "let's get on with it." More chemo is not always better. But I couldn't help thinking that the more I could tolerate the more likely it would kill the cancer. These drugs are toxic medications; in fact, they are called cytotoxic– meaning they are toxic to cells; they kill cells when the cells are dividing. All sorts of cells divide, but the cancer cells divide faster and are more likely to be killed. But the cells of the intestines also divide rapidly and so do the cells in the bone marrow that make white and red blood cells; the chemo would potentially kill many of them. And this would lead to the well know side effects of nausea, fatigue and susceptibility to infection. The hope was that the cancer cells that divide the fastest would also get killed faster and wouldn't grow back, while the normal healthy cells would recover.

Agustin seemed enthusiastic but I was anxious. I wanted to get started and kill the cancer cells right away, but I also felt dread and fear even as I was saying, "bring it on." Shouldn't we all have felt extremely sober and scared, after all I had Stage IV disease? Maybe he thought this was a problem he could solve. Maybe his enthusiasm was all about the chance to try something new with chemo. But it was my body the chemo would get pumped into and I could not consider it in the same way.

Finally, I said, "How will you know if it's working?"

Agustin explained, "Your cancer makes a lot of a cancer protein called CA-125, we can use that as the marker of response. We will track it and see if it goes down. And at the end we will repeat the scans."

Ovarian cancers are, in most cases, associated with a rise in CA-125. This is a protein that is associated with a particular genetic region and is detected by a simple blood test. But it is not used as a screening test. It can be elevated in women who do not have cancer (this called a false positive test) and it may not be elevated in women who do have cancer (this is a false negative test). To be a good screening test, it woold need to look for early disease and be shown to save lives by earlier diagnosis; CA-125 has not met that standard. For these reasons, it is not used as a screening test. But because the CA-125 in my blood was elevated, it could be used to see if the chemo was working. If the chemo worked, the CA-125 should come down.

The normal range for CA-125 is 0-35. Mine was 7,082. I was 200 times over normal. Could such a high level ever come down to normal? It was hard to imagine. How long did it take to get up to over 7,000 without me being aware of it? This was just another unanswerable question. In any event, the drop would need to be dramatic to get me to normal and even if it did get that low, there was no guarantee that it would stay low.

I headed off to the waiting area for the outpatient day hospital and put my name on the list to be called for my first chemo infusion. In the waiting area, people were chatting and reading. Some of them had no hair and wore some sort of bandana or hat, some left their bald heads uncovered, and I guessed at those who were wearing wigs knowing I would need to plan for hair loss also. Some were wearing masks for protection from infection knowing that their resistance was down. Some were restless and walked around and some were still. Most were with someone, a spouse, a friend, a child or in some cases a paid caregiver. They got coffee or tea at the hospitality cart. They picked up the magazines or newspapers left on side tables and thumbed through them. But for a waiting room with that many people it was unexpectedly quiet. Even cell phones seemed to be turned off. There was very little conversation and those talking with the person who brought them often spoke in whispers. People seemed afraid to look at each other. In any other situation they might not look so good, but almost all were able to walk on their own and that in itself was something to feel good about.

The nurse who called me into the day hospital was Filipino, less than five feet tall, bright eyed, with a childlike smile. She wore pink and purple nurse scrubs and had sparkly clips in her dark hair. She showed me to a bed and started explaining about the premeds to prevent nausea afterwards and to reduce allergic reactions. Thus began my 18 weeks of chemo with Imelda, my chemo nurse. Luck was with me that day. Imelda would be with me for those 18 weeks and what stretched into 16 months.

There were beds for chemo infusions and big chairs that looked like pedicure chairs. The beds were surrounded by curtains leaving just enough room for Jim to pull up a chair. Next to each was a metal pole to hang the saline bag and chemo bags, and there was a pump that measured and timed the infusion drip. Another machine recorded blood pressure and pulse at regular intervals. Imelda got the needle into a vein in my arm and threaded through the plastic catheter. As the needle was removed, she taped the plastic tubing to my arm and started the saline.

I was given four medications about one half hour before the chemo infusions were started. These were Kytril, Decadron, Pepcid, and Benadryl. Kytril and Decadron both helped to prevent nausea and vomiting. Pepcid controlled heartburn. Benadryl was to prevent allergic reactions and for sleep and it helped me relax and doze through chemo.

After half an hour to allow the premeds to work, Imelda returned. But now she had gloves on and a large paper smock over her purple scrubs to protect her from the chemo she was going to infuse directly into my veins. Three separate bags of liquid, one chemo drug infused at a time. Since this was my first infusion, she watched me closely. Although it is rare, some people break out in a rash and some spike high blood pressure. It was wait-and-see time. How would my body respond? My thoughts were a confusing mx of curiosity, fear, and prayer.

Physicians and nurses I knew stopped by. "You'll be fine," they all said, and I just hoped they were right. I had no anonymity but lots of encouragement and this felt like a good thing.

Over the next 18 weeks I got to know about Imelda's family, her boys who wanted to go to USC, her trips to Las Vegas, which according to Imelda, Filipinos loved to do. She showed me her picture with a tight short dress and her hair up, a very different look from the nurse scrubs and sparkly barrettes. She told me how she sang karaoke (which according to her all Filipinos did), how she got good deals in Vegas, her mom who was also a nurse (like a lot of Filipino women she said), how she came to be a nurse, what was on the nursing exams, how long she had been giving chemo, how Elisa and Erlinda the twin Filipino chemo nurses taught her to give chemo, Filipino food, the Filipino boxer Manny Pacquiao (who she said all Filipino women love), whether nurses should be in a union, and whether she could get free USC tuition benefits for her boys. She was chatty, and I grew to love her.

Every week when I showed up for chemo, I told the clerk at the desk that I wanted Imelda to be my chemo nurse. And every week that request was honored. I could see that other patients were also asking for their favorite nurses as well. This brought a great deal of continuity to the infusion process and it was very comforting to have a consistent relationship with one chemo nurse.

The three bags of chemo were slowly dripped in over a seven-hour period. We didn't leave until after dark. I walked to the car feeling like I had lost a day, but I was waiting for the effects of the chemo to hit me. "What will it feel like when it does?" I wondered.

I went home, ate a bit, watched TV, and went to bed early, still waiting for the chemo to hit me hard. The next morning, I went to work and while I could barely concentrate, it felt good to hold onto my normal routine. "Wow, not so bad," I thought.

Chapter 10: Holding Onto Normal

For some reason, unknown to the wisest of us, our department had several faculty members who developed unrelenting cancers. The Department of Preventive Medicine at USC has an outstanding national and international reputation for cancer epidemiology and cancer control research especially for cancers involving hormonal risk factors, such as breast, prostate and ovarian cancer. Conducting research on cancer does not keep anyone from getting it. One colleague developed breast cancer and was seemingly cured, then had a recurrence 13 years later. A colleague of 25 years developed glioblastoma, a brain tumor, and died from it. Another colleague developed a cutaneous lymphoma and died in his late fifties and another died from pancreatic cancer. One of my closest colleagues developed lymphoma. And now I was diagnosed with Stage IV ovarian cancer. Cancer is a common disease and nobody can assume they won't get it, but still faculty in our department had been saddened and even devastated by these deaths. News of my diagnosis spread quickly through the department. After the initial note to the institute faculty, I only personally told a few people and just trusted that the social network in my department would pass along the news.

"Why don't you just stay home and rest? It's OK – you have worked hard for a long time – now is the time to take care of yourself." These are words I heard from friends and colleagues and family. Why would I be clinging to work and the routines of going to my office, sitting in front of my computer, working on projects with students and colleagues, and even writing new grant proposals during what might have been the last years of my life? This made even less sense since prior to getting cancer, I had been contemplating early retirement to get away from the computer and the never-ending search for funding to continue my research. But hadn't I said the same words to others, thinking I was being helpful and offsetting any guilt they might have felt about loafing, or not working their way through it, or not being tough enough. It begs the question, "Why show up, why work when I may be dying?" As I tried to construct the answer for others (and myself) it did not seem like the obvious reaction. It was not the reaction that we often see in movies – the dramatic "travel-the-world-while-you-can" reaction; have an adventure, sky dive, or buy a sports car, and get out that bucket list. But being on chemo was incompatible with seeing the world and most other adventures, however small, that were on my bucket list. Although I don't even like the term "bucket list" because it conjured up frantically trying to fill in life experiences that had been postponed and ignored, but which became suddenly important near the end. How enjoyable was that?

It was also not the angry destructive reactions — get drunk or quit work. I remembered a Bert Reynolds movie, *The End.* After he was diagnosed, he tried to swim out in the ocean, too far to swim back. But then he changed his mind and bargained with God as he struggled to swim all the way back to shore.

It seemed humdrum to go to work when so little time might remain. So why did I do it?

The reason is simple. Cancer took so much away. I was tethered to the infusion clinic every week and there were days I was tethered to the sofa watching boring mid-day television, nonsense that fed into my fatigue and put me to sleep. Traveling and new adventures were incompatible with chemo but work at some level was not.

I cut my work schedule to three days a week in the office. I went to work, not because I was heroic or trying to prove something, and certainly not because I was actually still fully productive, but because I needed to go. I needed the people, the identity, and the routine. To avoid going would have let the cancer win and take too much away from me. Perseverating alone at home was an unwelcome alternative. One friend who also had cancer told me to expect to show up about half the time and to be about 25% productive, and she was right Still, I could not let cancer take that from me, I had already lost too much.

Cancer stole my focus. While I tried hard to think and focus, my scientific research questions retreated and the personal uncertainty questions advanced. How could I analyze data when numbers now made no sense, when it was hard to figure out simple things like a 20% tip for a meal or how much weight I had lost? My brain felt like a muddled soup due to the anemia and "chemo brain."

But yet, I needed to feel a connection with my pre-cancer self. The self that was a respected and productive faculty member and could be counted on to get things done well. The self that could get federally funded grants and conduct demanding research to reduce the burden of cancer, a disease I was now burdened by. The self that taught students and chaired dissertation committees and helped students figure out what research questions were important and how they could answer them. But also, the self that was part of a faculty group of extraordinary people who were committed to understanding more about serious diseases and generously helping each other with their work. Some department faculty had big reputations and were highly respected nationally and internationally and some were just starting out. I wanted to retain my place within this group.

After 30 years of working at one university, the faculty members and staff were my friends as well as my colleagues. And yet I was changed. I had crossed the invisible line and become one of the "subjects," one of those identified to be of research interest because I had developed one of the studied diseases. And more than anything, I wanted to not be on the other side of that line. But there was no way back. Yet by showing up at work, I felt I was straddling that line, walking the tightrope of that line. While one side, the familiar side, was my preference to fall into, I knew that I was falling off the other side of the tightrope where there was an unknown pit of an unknown future, the side with chemo and surgery and unpredictable results.

I began work on a NIH training grant that would offer continuing education for postdoctoral fellows. My plan was to write during the fall when I was on chemotherapy, put it aside for a while to recover after surgery, and then take it up again when I felt better to edit, finalize and submit in May. There was a lot of information to collect and put on tables and 20 pages of text to write. It seemed an ideal project for my abbreviated schedule and my chemo-addled brain that could not handle the analytic demands of more advanced technical research efforts right then.

After surgery and off of chemo, I read the document I wrote in the fall and was stunned by the incoherence of my text although fortunately the tables were completed largely due to the work of my colleague Marny, who picked up the burden of getting everything collected and organized. While I was aware of my mental limitations during chemo, particularly related to numerical calculations, I was unaware of the impact on my writing. And so, the editing plan was replaced with a serious rewrite before submission. It is not common knowledge, but all researchers know that less than 12% of NIH grant applications get funded. Alas, this was not one of them.

Chapter 11: Cycle 2 (weeks 4-6) — But It's Not Fun

It was week 4, the start of cycle 2 and all three drugs again. I was one-sixth done, and the road ahead looked long. I celebrated, but not really celebrated, my 62nd birthday during this cycle.

"Thousands of women have gotten through this and I will too," I said to myself. "Step by step, one foot in front of another. It's not so bad."

I did not want to have a port, a small plastic disc that sits under the skin, which connects to a catheter that then connects to a large vein internally close to the heart. The port can be used for blood draws and for chemo infusions. It is put in surgically and removed surgically. I had an aversion to getting one. It felt like one more thing to take care of and one more indication that I was sick. No, I really did not want a port.

My phlebotomist was a big guy, well over 6'2", big hands and broad like a football player. Pretty quickly I learned that he was both gentle and accurate and I would wait for him to do my blood draws. I was getting stuck a lot, a blood draw every week as well as a chemo stick. My veins needed to hold up and not collapse or get scarred and that meant I needed a good phlebotomist. Everyone on my team was important.

"Hey Princess, are you back again?" he asked.

"Yup – you'll see me every week," I told him.

"You know I'm a cancer survivor also," he said. "They didn't think I would beat it, but I am still here."

And thus began my blood draws that continued for seven years with that phlebotomist until he retired.

Blood monitoring is important, not just to check the CA-125 marker but more specifically to check levels of the white blood cells, red blood cells, and platelets since all were expected to drop from the chemo. Without the white blood cells, I would be susceptible to infections, without the red blood cells I would suffer fatigue from anemia, and without the platelets I could have impaired clotting. My bone marrow, where these cells are made, was getting beat up by the chemo, and while I wished I could control my blood cells, all I could do was hope. These cells needed to stay in the safe zone to have the next infusion of chemo. If they dropped too much, they might not give me chemo. And then what?

This time my nurse was Laurie. "How are you doing," she asked. "Still riding?"

Laurie and I both had horses and even though both of us had professions focused on cancer, we began every visit talking about our horses, and for a few minutes I was the horse owner and not the cancer patient.

"Yup," I replied, "I am still riding and jumping courses – not big stuff – actually my horse, Santana, can jump big but he's lazy and I never got to the point of jumping more than three feet and even less now. But it feels so good. There is nothing like it."

I had questions written down so I wouldn't forget to ask. "I have heartburn and a constant cough that seems not to respond to cough drops or syrup. I don't have a fever or feel like I have an infection."

"It's acid reflux," replied Lilia my nurse practitioner, as she wrote out a prescription for stronger antacid pills to take every day.

The effects of chemo were starting to build. Mouth sores and what my friend described as a " shredded esophagus" kept me from eating anything acidic or dense – even oatmeal was too much. I had read the nutritional guides for a balanced diet for people on chemo, the problem was that I could not eat those foods.

A few minutes later Agustin entered the exam room. "Look," he said, "your CA-125 has dropped a lot. It is now 2132. It's down by two thirds." Agustin seemed jubilant like the smart kid in the class who just aced the exam.

It was more than I had dared hope for. And I knew it might not keep going down at this rate. But there was no question, cancer cells were dying, the chemo was working, and I said a little prayer of thanks.

"Is the node in your armpit any smaller?" he asked.

I had been obsessively checking it in the intervening three weeks. "Yes," I said, "it feels smaller to me. I'm pretty sure it is smaller." Why couldn't I say it was definitely smaller? It was and I knew it but I was afraid to voice it: what if I was wrong and it had not shrunk at all?

He checked it, closing his eyes and mentally measuring it again. "It is smaller, definitely."

Next, he asked, "how's the hair?"

"It's thin, its falling out, it feels prickly. Pretty soon I will need a hat or something," I said.

I asked a few questions I had written out in the prior three weeks. Then off I went back to see Imelda to start cycle 2, all three drugs again. I knew I had a long day to get all of them infused.

Another nurse I didn't know was helping that day. "No port?" she asked.

"No," I replied, "I wanted to see if I could do without a port. I ride horses and I don't want to have to be careful of a port. If my veins don't hold up, I'll have to get one but I want to see if I can do without."

"It's so much easier," she said in response. "You know you can do the blood draws and the infusions through it."

"I know, I would just prefer not to have it," I said. "Easier for her or for me?" I thought. I felt myself digging in. I had few choices and the choices I could make I did not intend to relinquish.

"Doctor Garcia doesn't always use ports unless it is necessary, if we can't get into a vein or if the patient can't handle needle sticks," Imelda said in my defense. We both wanted this nurse to leave.

The other nurse looked dubious, either due to my decision to not have a port or because I was riding horses while on chemo, I couldn't tell which. When she left, Imelda and I both rolled our eyes as she inserted the needle to start the saline and give the pre-meds. The Benadryl started to take hold and I began to doze.

A while later, my friend Susan came by to visit. Our offices were nearly next to each other and two floors directly above the infusion clinic. She is both one of the smartest and most compassionate people I know. I could say anything to her about cancer and chemo and she was not afraid to talk about it. She listened to my fears and my optimism without judging either. We shared thoughts on physical challenges, and mental tricks for dealing with all of the changes as well as names of massage therapists and comfortable shoes. She took a break from work every week for 18 weeks, came down to the clinic and stayed for a chat during my infusions, then she returned to her office two floors above and went back to work.

A short time later, my friends Sue and Yvonne also came by. I had worked with Yvonne for 30 years and with Sue for 12 years. Sue, Yvonne, and Susan, were regular visitors for that 18-week chemo marathon. My friends Kay, Lourdes, and Kathleen came by interrupting their work day and staying for a short chat. Other doctors stopped by as they also were in the clinic to monitor their own patients. Jim and Imelda were there every week and through the entire infusion even though it took many hours. It could have been a lonely experience, and many patients seemed to get through it very much alone. It was probably unusual, to have this number of visitors during infusions and I came to realize this was an advantage of being treated only two floors below my own office. Friends would tell stories and jokes and stifle laughs as I was getting infused with toxic medications. We talked about anything and everything even those Kardashians. I was grateful for their company and so was Jim. Yvonne would laugh when she stopped by, presumably to give Jim a break so he could take a walk or go get coffee, but in fact, he stayed to chat while they were there and left for coffee only after they left and I started dozing again.

Chapter 12: Living Through Chemo: Eating, Pooping, Stiffness and Aches

Many people have an outdated image of chemotherapy. They expect the treatment to have horrific side effects. It is no picnic, and there were some very difficult days, but for me, it was not horrific. Many of the side effects that were not controlled 10 or 20 years ago, are now well controlled due to anti-nausea and anti-vomiting drugs (antiemetic drugs) given before every infusion.

Chemotherapy works by killing cells when they are dividing. The cells lining the intestines divide every 2 to 4 days. This is not as fast as cancer cells but it is still fast enough for some of these cells to be killed by the chemo. The digestive system is basically a long tube made up of mouth, esophagus, stomach, small intestine, large intestine, rectum and anus. The chemo hits the cells lining the digestive system pretty hard just because they are dividing fast. This means the digestive system needs special care from top to bottom during chemo.

By the second day after my first chemo infusion, I felt the initial effects of chemo. Eating became hard for me right away. Stomach and intestinal upset and the heartburn kept me from eating normally. My sense of taste was also altered. Everything tasted salty or metallic. Water tasted like salt water and tea tasted like it came right out of the Pacific Ocean. But the problem wasn't solely with taste. It was also the texture; I could not swallow anything dense or fibrous. I lost a few pounds on the weeks that I had the carboplatin, but I was able to gain it back again in the weeks that I had only Taxol so I reasoned that the carboplatin was the one I was having trouble with.

Chemo caused a persistent irritation of my esophagus due to acid reflux. The esophageal irritation led to a cough and a scratchy throat. I was given a prescription strength version of Prilosec called Protonics. Taking this medication every evening throughout my chemo helped the acid reflux and stopped the cough, but I still could not eat a normal diet.

I did not want to eat raw foods because my immune system was weakened and I did not want to get any food-borne infections. I was also concerned about anemia and that my red blood cells might go so low that it would be dangerous to get chemotherapy. I was told that iron rich foods would not save me from anemia while I was on chemo, yet I thought it was worth a try to eat more spinach, lamb chops and fillet mignon, which were iron rich but fairly soft. Iron supplements can cause constipation and so I avoided them also.

Due to mouth sores, I could not eat anything acidic such as tomatoes, orange juice, and salad dressing. My eating habits had to change. Thus began the soft and bland diet. Milkshakes with tofu, yogurt, bananas, and vanilla ice cream became my go-to food for 18 weeks. For dinner: butternut squash soup, yogurt, cheese and a scrambled egg and sometimes pasta with butter and cheese. I needed to find food I could comfortably eat and that took some experimentation. This persisted through 18 weeks of chemo.

Constipation turned out to be a big problem. It seemed that whatever I ate was just not coming out the other end. And then I saw that the toilet bowl was filled with bright red blood. I had a routine colonoscopy five months before I was diagnosed so I was pretty sure it was hemorrhoids and not something more sinister. Yet, I was afraid that losing blood while on chemo would hasten anemia and I did not want that either. Mostly I did not want anything to interrupt the chemo that was my lifeline to eradicate the cancer.

Agustin referred me to a gastro-intestinal (GI) surgeon. I dreaded this appointment because I was afraid he might want to operate on my hemorrhoids and delay my cancer treatment. I began to regret admitting that I was having this problem.

I did not recognize the nurses in the GI clinic, and they did not recognize me. I felt like a "typical patient" and it made me realize how really cared for I felt with my familiar oncology nurses. With them, it was smiles and chitchat and support. In this GI clinic I was just a patient with hemorrhoids and cancer – not a great description I must admit. Gratefully, the doctor did an exam and concluded that nothing should be done – the chemo took priority. He suggested Benefiber and more Benefiber. I could do that and I was grateful for his response.

Thus began the Benefiber, stool softeners, Preparation H and warm Epson salts baths every day. Eating and pooping were going to be a challenge, something so normal that now needed to be managed. Finally, all of the measures I took worked and the hemorrhoid bleeding nearly stopped, at least enough so that it stopped worrying me. This felt like one more problem solved.

*

Shortly after my treatment started, I needed to figure out how to reduce and relieve anxiety and to relax my body. Fight or flight is a natural response. To muster combative energy or to run away. But neither of these were good responses to cancer.

My solution was Epson salt baths and yoga. Yoga is not my favorite form of exercise. I am not flexible, graceful, or meditative and while I had tried it from time to time, it was not something that had been a regular part of my life. But I needed something I could do to keep the anxiety from creeping into every muscle and fiber in my body causing me to be physically frozen and unable to move.

My body felt achy. I don't know if this was due to tension held in every muscle and ligament or if chemo had that effect. In a few weeks I felt like I could barely move my head from side to side. I began to take warm Epson salts baths twice a day during chemo. I soaked in our deep old bathtub with hot water up to my neck. While I was soaking, I was not able to put cancer out of my mind. I would go over and over my progress. The baths gave me a time to do the "worry-work". What exactly is "worry-work"? It was a half hour in the morning and in the evening to sort through my thoughts. It was a time to reflect on my fear and think about what my future might be. It was a time to think about what I would want to do if it became clear that my lifetime would be short or long. It was a time to think about what I needed to do tomorrow and the next day – and what I needed to do when I got out of that tub. It was time to take stock of how my body really felt and whether my feet still had sensation and how they were tingling from neuropathy. It was a time to wash the little itty bit of hair I had left. And this is the way it is with cancer. It was also a peaceful time, almost meditative and a time to recenter myself on my three words: gratitude, integrity and determination. As the water cooled, I added more hot water and steamed myself until Jim came in to see what was taking me so long. The baths helped to relax my mind and kept me from falling into an emotional rathole.

On the second floor of my house, with an ancient VCR player and my GAIAM Rodney Yee VHS yoga tapes, I would do my best to stretch and strengthen. The "Sun Salutation" is a lovely series of yoga movements that stretched and strengthened many of my core and large muscles and yet it was easy enough for me to practice however awkwardly.

What did yoga do for me? It was a way of saying to myself, "I am OK, my body is my own, it doesn't belong to the cancer, regardless of what this cancer is doing, right now I am in control of how I am functioning, and right now I am doing yoga to help me stay strong." It was a way of saying that I was fighting back to keep my body healthy, but fighting back in a non-aggressive way that was gentle to my body. I did yoga stretches at random times even if it was waiting for a few minutes while I was boiling an egg or making a cup of tea. There were days I was unable to stand on one foot or to hold downward dog for any length of time even though it is considered to be a resting pose. Yoga is not a competitive sport so whether I was doing better or worse from day to day, it did not matter. It was all about using movement to help me feel better. Yoga got me off of the sofa. It was a way for me to move, release my anxiety, make my tensed-up muscles relax, focus on something other than fear, and force myself to simply breathe.

Baths and yoga were about self-care and about taking control over what I could control. They were about easing the fear in my anxious mind and moving forward with focused actions that helped me deal with the difficult journey.

Chapter 13: Cycle 3 (Weeks 7-9) — Climbing a Mountain

"How have you been doing? Any problems?" asked Lilia my nurse practitioner.

My hair was gone and I felt tired and sore.

"Are you still working?" she asked.

"Yes, three days a week," I responded, "I think it's better for me than sitting home. I don't feel terrible but I know my workdays are not highly productive either. But still, it feels better to go to work."

But I didn't want to talk about my work schedule. The question burning in my mind was a number. What was the CA-125 level this cycle? It would tell me if the first cycle was a fluke or if it was continuing to drop. I was anxious to know that number.

Lilia pulled up my laboratory results on the computer. "Your CA-125 dropped again. You are now at 193," Lilia said.

"That's a big drop," I said almost speechless. Proportionally it was a huge drop and I could have calculated that percent in my head at one point, but all I could come up with that day was "a big drop." Sometimes "big" is a better description than an exact percent.

I was surprised it had dropped that much because I really did not expect it, I expected it to start leveling out. I began to think I might make it through after all. The chemo was doing its job, I was doing my job, and I began to feel like I was winning.

What does it feel like to be on chemo? When my children were little and I needed to attend a meeting on the east coast, I would try to minimize my time gone. I can recall a few trips when I would go to work for a full day, then go home for dinner and bedtime with the kids, then go to the airport for a red eye flight to Washington DC, arrive early in the morning and go to a meeting all day, then take the evening flight home sleeping on the airplane. My car would have been parked at the airport for less than 24 hours. Sometimes I would drive home, often feeling wired. But when I got home and fell into bed, I would not be able to fall asleep. Early the next morning I would get up to get the kids off to school and I went off to work. By the time I got to work, I struggled to concentrate, I could not think, my balance was probably a bit off, my reaction time was probably slowed. At lunch time I would close my office door and lie down on a mat in my office to catch a quick nap. That is what chemotherapy felt like on a daily basis in terms of mental reactions. During chemo I often used the mat in my office to take a short nap to get through a full day.

Well, at least I could read novels, I thought. But after spending a long time reading the same pages over and over again and still not knowing what those pages said, I realized that I couldn't even concentrate on that. Cancer thoughts, the "what ifs," were taking over and invading my mind like a noisy neighbor who I could not get rid of and could not ignore.

On long nights, I could not fall asleep and I just stared at the ceiling all night asking questions I could not answer and by morning, I was exhausted. I could handle my anxiety during the distractions of the day but at night it hit me. I kept going over and over the same questions and possibilities and there were no answers. It was not helpful and it went nowhere, but I couldn't seem to put it out of my mind and get to sleep. "I need something to help me sleep," I told Lilia.

A low dose sleeping pill was the answer most nights. It seemed that, on balance, it was healthier to do that than to be exhausted from no sleep. It was a trade-off that I wish I had been able to handle another way. But I had to accept that the unwelcome interlopers of worry and anxiety would visit me in the middle of the night and stay till morning, sitting like a troll on my pillow and whispering questions and uncertainties all night long. The sleeping pill shut those goons out.

At the end of week nine I was at the half way point. It was like climbing a mountain and getting to the summit. Now it was just a matter of going down the other side without falling. "Half done, half done, half done, all downhill from here."

Chapter 14: And Now a Word About Hair

I knew I would lose my hair and everyone either wanted to tell me that I would lose it or ask me if I would lose it. "You will lose your hair," Agustin said and so did the consulting physician, the phlebotomist, the PET scan tech, and my friend with breast cancer and my friend with lymphoma.

"Will you lose your hair?" other friends asked.

"Yes, no doubt. Small price to pay to regain my life."

"Will you get a wig?"

"I don't think so."

"Why not?" some said with curiosity and maybe some horror.

"Scratchy, uncomfortable, hot, fake-looking, don't want to take care of it," I said. Some of my friends who had been on chemo rarely wore the wigs they bought.

"I am going to donate my hair," said another friend with beautiful long hair.

"That's a kind thing to do," I said, "somebody will want it very much."

"What will you do?"

"Scarves, hats – I'll figure it out." I was cavalier at the start.

Some women with great bone structure and enormous eyes look stunning and gazelle-like with no hair. But I was pretty sure I would not look that way.

"How can I help?" my brother asked.

"Let's go buy hats," I said.

We went to Broken Horn where there were rows of cowboy hats, wool felt hats, straw hats, black and tan hats with wide brims, and smaller hats like those worn by female country singers. There were also baseball hats with rhinestones and emblems from sports teams and motorcycle clubs.

I picked out a straw cowgirl hat. My brother picked out a baseball hat; it was white with embroidered grey wings and a pink heart and rhinestones. "Really?" I thought, "does my brother see me completely differently than I see myself?" We bought them both.

The first few weeks of chemo, no hair fell out, and I began to think maybe it wouldn't. I was getting through this, going to work, and some people could not even tell I had cancer. But one day I noticed that there was hair all over my black office chair. I ran my fingers through my hair and my hand came away covered with hair. The reality of hair loss hit me. This was really happening. I was losing my hair and it was going fast.

I called Cesare my Lebanese hairdresser. "Come today," he said. Pretty quickly I went from blond chin length hair to a grey-roots pixie cut for another few weeks as the shower drain caught hair every day until all of that hair was gone.

As I looked in the mirror I could see more and more of my scalp and every day I looked older and older until there were only wisps of grey hair around the edges. My head felt cold all of the time. I hated to look in the mirror. Who was the old woman looking back? Every day I felt less and less attractive and every day I had to say to myself, "It is just for a while – it shows the chemo is killing some hair growth cells just like it is killing the cancer cells."

"Get a wig," said another patient with ovarian cancer who I met during chemo. "I have been through losing my hair over and over again with recurrences – I don't think my hair will ever come back, it's the only way I can function and pass as normal."

"Pass as normal." That's interesting and appealing. A wig is a way to pass as healthy – to hide the cancer, to not have to explain, to not stand out when all you want to do is to fit in, to be normal and avoid seeing the sympathy or even the pity of others.

I had cancer, I was on chemo, and my hair fell out. That was the reality and maybe I could disguise this. But why do that and be uncomfortable with a wig? But like others, I was also avoiding notice, with my hats, especially my brother's choice, the flashy pink heart, grey wings and rhinestones. But at times it felt like I was trying to hide a dirty secret.

My friend Marilyn, with breast cancer was also on chemo. She taught junior high school students. She didn't try to hide her hair loss and even took it a step further. She told her classroom of kids that she was on chemo and losing her hair, and then she took off her hat and showed them her balding head. It did not look pretty and I could not imagine doing that even with my college students.

"How did they react?" I asked.

"They have been amazingly considerate," she said. "Now when I say – stay away and sit in the back of the room if you have a cold, they don't question it. They show their concern and are behaving better."

But I worked in a cancer center, and if my colleagues couldn't handle seeing me without hair, that would be a pretty sad statement about them.

Another friend had her husband shave her head. To shave or not to shave that is the question. Why not? But then again, why? I was going to cover it up anyway so why did I need to shave off the bits of hair that remained on my head. It looked awful with sprigs of hair here and there, but the hair that stuck out a bit around the edges of my hat looked OK, at least to me, so I kept what was left.

My daughter's friends Tina and Morgen both wore their hair in short spikey cuts. "I can't wait till my hair is as long as yours," I said and we all laughed. "I work hard to get my hair like this," said Tina "it really takes a lot of fussing and product." Even short spikey hair looked like long hair now.

When friends asked what they could do; I said, "buy me a hat", which they did: cowgirl hats, baseball hats, ski hats, English caps, wide brimmed beach hats, and soft jersey beanies.

I had no idea how to tie my head in a scarf and despite watching YouTube videos, the scarf would slide around and not stay put. As the scarf slipped it fell over and covered one eye; a man I had worked with for a long time teased that it looked like I was going for the "pirate look," which unfortunately was true.

Nobody tells you that you will lose hair everywhere. I lost the hair on my arms, my legs, and every place else. Hair is hair, eyebrows and eyelashes - gone. Losing eyebrows is surprisingly disconcerting. I looked like humpty dumpty.

Laila told me that one of her patients had refused Taxol because she did not want to have hair loss and I couldn't help but fear for anyone who would forego optimal treatment for the sake of hair. When I looked in the mirror, I was startled; there was nothing pretty about it. I certainly didn't want to look like a cancer patient but it had to be tolerated, and I decided that any way I dealt with it, whether it was wigs or hats, would be the right way.

My son, David, asked how to explain this to my three-year old grandson. "Well – just tell him that GoGo (what my grandchildren call me) is on medicine that is very strong because she got sick for a while. The medicine made her hair fall out, but it will come back soon. Tell him this does not happen with most medicine but just with this special and very strong medicine that GoGo had to take."

Would my little grandson even notice? But one day I didn't have a hat on and when he looked at me, I could see the question on his face. "Does my hair look different?" I asked him. He nodded. He came behind my chair and his small hands very gently felt my head and the hair that was left. I waited to see what would happen next. But that little touch was enough to satisfy his curiosity. He went back to playing. Tinkertoys were far more interesting.

Chapter 15: Cycle 4 (Weeks 10-12) —My Stomach Says "Enough"

Fluid was building up underneath my fingernails and they were oozing and sore. I was afraid they were going to fall off as my hair had done. I didn't expect the chemo to work its way all the way to my fingernails, and the thought of my fingernails falling off felt repulsive.

"What can I do about this?" I asked Laurie showing her my mushy nails.

"Soak them in dilute hydrogen peroxide," she said.

I tried to force myself to consider my nails as I did my hair. This was a small price to pay. That was how I dealt with the side effects of chemo. Every unexpected small and big chemo effect was "just a small price to pay to get my life back." But still I hated my mushy nails and I hated having yet another effect that made me feel every day more and more like a sack of sickness.

When Agustin came into the exam room he joked, "I hear your fingers are falling off."

"Not funny," I said, knowing that he could get away with this dark humor with me and probably wouldn't say this to most of his patients.

"Hydrogen peroxide," he said. On his list of problems from seeing patients all day, this was clearly low on his list. And he was right.

The neuropathy which had started as numbness and tingling in my feet, like pins and needles was now beginning to feel like I had marbles in my shoes and some days it felt quite painful. Neuropathy is one of those expected and hard-to-control side effects of chemo. While many patients focus on hair loss, neuropathy is actually a much more significant problem. It was progressing to pain that caused me to jerk my feet as though getting stuck with needles. Some people end up in a wheel chair due to the neuropathy because they cannot walk when their feet are in pain. Some people fall because they cannot feel their own feet. For some it never goes away even after they have been off chemo for years.

"Try L-Carnetine," Agustin said, "you can get it at the health-food store. There is a clinical trial that uses about four times the listed dose to see if it helps neuropathy. You can try it even if you aren't on the trial." He also gave me a prescription for another medication, Gabapentin as well. My medications were mounting up and that in itself was unsettling, so I decided to try the L-Carnetine first.

"I had a bloody nose a few times this cycle," I told him. I knew this was due to the bevacizumab, an anti-angiogenesis drug that interferes with growth of new blood vessels. Because tumors require a blood supply to grow, the tumor itself stimulates blood vessel growth to feed the interior of the tumor. Bevacizumab works to prevent the growth of these blood vessels and thus it is starving the tumor of a blood supply. This is a newer medication and supplements the regular chemo medications. But it also caused my face to be flushed, which made me look healthier than I was. It caused bleeding when I brushed my teeth and an occasional bloody nose. "Small price to pay," I said yet again.

I was staying away from crowds and sick friends or runny-nose grandkids to try to avoid getting an infection. I knew my immunity had to be down with low white blood cells from the chemo. My red blood cells were also low, and this caused fatigue. My horseback riding had deteriorated to walking around for a half hour and letting my horse, Santana, wander. To the extent he thought about it, he probably wondered whether I was asleep in the saddle. I could not feel my feet in the stirrups and had no idea if I was keeping my heels down in what should be good form.

My entire digestive system felt assaulted, starting with my lips that had developed sores making it even harder to eat. Any sort of acid from a tomato to a pineapple slice would send me to the refrigerator to grab milk to stifle the pain. The heartburn and the metallic and salty taste of most foods made eating a chore. Normally, I like to shop for good food, I like to cook, and I like to eat so this was way out of my normal relationship with food. Food for me is a source of enjoyment and a way to build community and family; it is for celebration and for solitude. Preparing food is not a thoughtless activity that I just rush through. Even though I had wanted to lose ten pounds before I was diagnosed, when I lost those ten pounds on chemo I found that I wanted that ten pounds back, more because it was an unintended loss rather than that I needed them.

"Your CA-125 is down to 37.6," Agustin said, "it's essentially in the normal zone." I could hardly believe it. It had dropped over 7000 units. I knew I was lucky; this does not always happen. I was at the half-way point. The next nine weeks would be insurance – maybe the bulk of the cancer cells had been killed, but every last one of those cells needed to be killed to keep the cancer from coming back. It was like killing ants in the kitchen, you think you have them all and then you notice movement and see there are lots of them still crawling around. It's hard to get them all.

And then, during Cycle 4 a few days after having all three drugs, the vomiting began. Vomiting from chemo is a very different kind of experience than food poisoning, flu, or any other stomach upset or nausea I have ever felt. It is not that there was something in my stomach causing the problem, it was my stomach itself that was the problem. My stomach felt cold, hard, and metallic and I guessed the platinum in the carboplatin made it feel that way. I imagined it felt like being poisoned.

The thing about chemo is that vomiting is sudden. All of a sudden the urgency to vomit is so strong that I had to run for the toilet. Even after whatever was in my stomach was now in the toilet or the pot on the floor next to the sofa, my stomach was searching in that empty sack to find anything else to expel. Finding nothing, my stomach tried to turn itself inside out and exit my body, like it was trying to flee the poison raining down on it.

Vomiting was harsher than I imagined it would be, and it came on me unexpectedly after not having this problem during the first nine weeks. Vomiting quickly becomes dry heaves to the point of exhaustion. Drinking a little bit of water to take the acid taste out of my mouth just started the heaving again. It went on for hours. I could not move. Any movement would start the dry heaves again and so I lay on the sofa trying to keep still or sleep, while watching daytime TV. My dog Jackson looked at me mournfully and I looked at him in exactly the same way.

Jim called Lilia, and she called back right away. She prescribed Compazine and little by little the vomiting left as unannounced as it had come. I was weak, but back to my milkshakes.

It lasted three days and it only happened on the week I had carboplatin. I only had two more carboplatin infusions to go, so even if it happened again, and I dreaded that, I knew I could get through it.

Chapter 16: In the Dirt

In 2003, at 55 years old, I bought a horse. It was late in life to do this but I had wanted a horse since I was a child and it felt like I had reached the now-or-never point. Santana was a seven-year-old dark-bay Hanoverian. At 17 hands he was a big horse. Some horses have a gait that causes every step to slam the rider's vertebrae and some horses glide. Santana glided. His gaits were incredibly smooth and his stride was long. He had been poorly trained and had the reputation as an "incremental learner," that is, he needed to learn small lessons over long periods of time. I soon learned that he had athletic ability that had not even been tapped. While he could jump a four-foot jump, I was satisfied at two to three feet high. By the time I was diagnosed in 2010, he was reformed and we were jumping those small fences.

When I was diagnosed, I wanted to hold onto everything that was a normal part of my life including riding. Santana helped me get through a hard time. I started chemo and I continued to jump over small jumps. But with chemo, my balance was off. I was wobbly which is a bad thing on a big horse. I had neuropathy in my feet so that I had a hard time feeling the stirrups. And most of all, chemo gave me anemia and fatigue so that my endurance was diminished. If I broke something that needed surgical repair, the bevacizumab would interfere with healing. So, I needed to be especially careful.

Jumping fences can be tricky. You need to be straight and well balanced. You also need to "see a distance" to the fence, how close or far you were from the fence, and regulate the horses stride length and pace to meet it just right. The take off point can't be too close or too far away. As the chemo built up, my ability to perceive how far away I was and how many strides it would take to get to the jump was ebbing away. On a beautiful fall day, Santana and I parted company over a fence and I found myself in the dirt. As I lay on the ground, looking up at the sky, worried faces crowded around me. "I'm ok – Just give me a minute to catch my breath," I said. The rule in riding is, "get back on and do it again," so that you fix whatever you did wrong.

"You came into the jump unbalanced; do you want to try it again?" a friend said.

"Yes, but when I am done with chemo. Not now," I managed to say. I had to face reality and lying there in the dirt was a good place to do that. That was it. There would be no more jumping until after chemo and, depending on how things went, maybe never again.

Still, as the chemo built up and the anemia increased, I continued to ride. It was a diversion from thinking about cancer and my treatment. But sometimes even on horseback, nothing could blot out the worry. I rode all through 18 weeks of hard chemo and the 6 weeks off chemo before surgery even though this often meant nothing more than walking Santana after he had been tired out by a younger, healthier rider.

Riding made me get out of the house, to get outdoors, to groom my horse, clean my saddle, and do normal barn chores. It helped my healing. It gave me small goals and it strengthened my body and my mind.

I made a promise to Santana that if he took care of me through treatment then he would have a home for life. He would not get sold and would retire in a field in his old age where my friend Terri would take care of him. He kept his end of the deal and I kept mine. Santana is now 25 years old. He lives in a field in Northern California with a herd of retired horses that regard him as the "Boss." He is living out his older years eating and lazing around with his new buddies, probably exactly what he prefers. Promises were kept. He is happy and I am alive.

Chapter 17: Cycle 5 (Weeks 13-15) — The Magic Number

I was counting down the weeks. Six weeks to go. I was on the downward slope and headed for the end. Soon this would be over.

My appointment was five days after Thanksgiving, one of my favorite holidays when I usually blow out the kitchen, cooking everything, having people over and all of us eating until we just lay on the floor and talked about going for a walk. But this year I had a modified meal, cream of chicken soup.

"What is my count now," I asked obsessively charting my CA-125 levels (and in fact I did have a chart).

"It's 24.8" Lilia said. It had dropped below the red line on my chart separating elevated, above 35, from normal, below 35.

The L-Carnitine seemed to be working. My feet had stopped getting worse and seemed to be getting a bit better. I had less stabbing pain although the pins and needles continued, but I could feel my feet again.

"You need to go see Dr. Muderspach," said Agustin. I had not seen Laila, my gynecological oncology surgeon, since she did my uterine biopsy.

"Do I need to have surgery now?" I asked Agustin. It had been in the back of my mind all through chemo. But with the focus on chemo, I had stopped thinking about surgery. Surgery for ovarian cancer is usually done before chemo. But, as in my case, when the cancer has spread out of the abdomen, it is done after chemo or sometimes the chemo is split with half before and half after surgery.

It just seemed sensible to get all of these organs out – ovaries, fallopian tubes, uterus, omentum, some lymph nodes After all, I was 62 years old, God was not going to bless me with another pregnancy nor did I want Her to. That I knew for sure. So, I was ready to get rid of these parts, and good riddance to them. With cancer, I had the overwhelming urge like most people, to just get this foreign invader cut out of my body.

"Probably – but that is Laila's expertise, you need to talk to her," he said and then once again, I was off to the infusion clinic and Imelda.

I had taken to wearing an old sweatshirt to chemo visits – a pale green one that said "Alaska" in blue on it from a trip five years before. I felt cold all of the time especially in the infusion room. They had warmed blankets for patients and I would often need a few of them to feel warm during the infusion. I would cover myself up to the neck, wear my knit hat and my sweatshirt and try to doze through the infusion. Some patients looked like they were maintaining business appropriate dress – what you would normally wear to go to the doctor, neat and put together. My only thought was comfort and warmth. I looked like I was ready to go camping, bundled up in sweats and a hat.

Three days after the infusion of the three drugs on cycle 5, I again had vomiting and it felt more severe than in cycle 4. The Compazine did not seem to help so Jim called Lilia again to see if there was anything else that might help. She prescribed another drug that Jim picked up at the pharmacy. This gave me two medications to take at home for breakthrough nausea and vomiting. They were prochlorperazine (also called Compazine) taken on a schedule to get ahead of bad nausea and ondansetron HCL for worse nausea if the Compazine was not sufficient

In my chemo brain haze I needed to label all of my pills to keep them straight since the drug names only added to the confusion. I had taken no pills prior to cancer, but now I had a medicine cabinet full of pills that I labeled "for reflux," "for bad vomiting," "for really bad vomiting," "for sleep," and "for neuropathy." This time the vomiting again lasted intensely for a few miserable days. Weak, shaky and hungry, I got to the other side.

I made an appointment with Laila to talk about surgery. "Your response to the chemo has been exceptional, but you need surgery," she said. "We need to do everything we can to keep it from coming back. It's a big surgery. It will take several hours. I think I can do this robotically with several small incisions but I will know more after the scans."

Laila let me know what was ahead. "You need another CT and PET scan so we can see how much the cancer has shrunk. You need to be off the bevacizumab for six weeks before surgery. So, let's schedule surgery for mid February. After surgery I want you to stay off work for 6 weeks and off your horse too. I mean it, no work and no riding. You will heal better and faster if you do that. You need to put in for temporary disability now to cover you while you recover."

"Ok," I agreed, "I want it all out." At some level it was so easy to say and so different from my attitude before cancer when I thought I would exit this world with all of my body parts intact, taking some unearned pride in keeping every part of myself together. But now that was no longer important.

When I think back on conversations with Laila, I realize again how lucky I was. For most women, finding the right surgeon, getting an appointment, meeting and trying to establish rapport with a surgeon is often one of the major challenges of seeking care for cancer. Patients are already afraid and in a state of shock at the diagnosis and then they need to go into a medical system that they don't understand searching for the best surgeon, calling friends and doctors, getting referrals, and putting blind trust in professional summaries on the internet. They often go into surgery having met their surgeon only once or twice and the second time is often when they are getting wheeled into the operating room.

What is the solution for the discomfort patients often feel in the medical setting? How can they participate and interact more effectively with their medical providers? While there is probably no way to quickly become comfortable and familiar, some help is available.

- Some hospitals provide patient navigators, social workers or advocates who can help coordinate care and even go to appointments with patients. A good friend or family member, especially someone with some medical knowledge can be helpful.

- Ask for one consistent chemo nurse.

- Ask each person's name when you meet them, write it down with a description and talk with your nurses by name.

- Learn about your treatment and write down your questions so that you can efficiently ask for the help and information you need. Appointment times are short. Be clear about what you are asking.

- Keep a list of side effects that you experience and how long and severe they were. This helps you and is appreciated by providers.

- Ask for what you need, don't wait for busy providers to figure it out all the while you are feeling neglected and they are feeling unappreciated. Try to keep the communication positive even if you feel terrible.

All of these may help to overcome the divide between you and your providers.

"How old is your oldest child?" I asked Laila. "

He is 22, he just finished at UCLA," she replied.

"Well then we have known each other longer than that," I said. "We met before you were pregnant with him. I completely trust you on this."

Chapter 18: A Good Dog

In 2010, Jackson was my constant companion as I lay on the sofa, in a chemo funk, watching TV and willing myself to get up and be productive – and failing that test of self-willpower. But, Jackson didn't care. He was more than willing to lie next to the sofa for hours with my arm hanging over the side and hand buried in his thick black fur, only raising his head when the scratching and patting subsided.

He was five years old when Jim and I rescued him in 2007, the unwanted dog in a divorce. He was the husband's dog until he either moved out or was thrown out, and then the wife took Jackson to the pound. Ninety pounds of black Labrador Retriever, looking like he had a few extra vertebrae that caused his long back to sag. But his head was pure lab, big, with expressive brown eyes and floppy ears. He had been at the pound a long time and his time was running out, nobody seemed to want him. When we told the volunteer we were looking for a Lab, she quickly gave him a bath and tracked us down as we meandered along peering into cage after cage. She was determined that we would give him a chance.

"I believe in this dog," she said.

I liked her choice of words. I could tell right away that Jim was ready to take him home.

Once we got him in the car, he slept all of the way to our house, seemingly glad to be rid of the chaos and noise of the pound. We soon learned that eating and sleeping were his major interests in life. We began to call him the "greeter" and sometimes we called him "the butler." He was always appropriate. He was like the nanny dog in Peter Pan; children and babies could climb over him, dress him up, examine his teeth and ears, put him in their pillow forts, and he would be a quiet victim to their imaginary play. Not a watchdog, he welcomed friends and strangers alike.

Jackson was an old soul. By the time I got cancer he was eight. How much do dogs understand when their people are going through a hard time? Some people think their dogs understand their fear and grief and incapacity. There is even research showing that dogs can smell cancer in the urine of a person with cancer. I am not sure that was true of Jackson, but maybe it was. But I can say, he was with me always when I was home and I can say that he helped me get through. Cancer is a lonely experience even with family and friends who at some point need to continue their other responsibilities. But Jackson had no responsibilities other than to stick by me and that's what he did and that is what I needed.

Chapter 19: Cycle 6 (Weeks 16-18) — Don't Move the Finish Line

It was the last cycle. My marker was down to 19.2.

"You are doing great," Jim said, "almost done."

"I know, but I feel like I have aged 30 years in the last few months. I feel like I am 90 years old. I feel worn-out, achy, hairless and weak."

"Well, when it's done you will start feeling better, you'll get back to normal. You will age backwards and start feeling younger."

I could only hope that would happen. I knew this had not been easy for him either. He had never been really sick and he felt so uncomfortable in medical settings, with the needles, the jargon that he didn't understand, blood, pumps, chemo, officious people, and even the smell of hospitals. And seeing me going from a competent, healthy woman to a foggy headed, aging, progressively sicker woman wasn't a happy experience.

But he liked my medical team Agustin, Laila, Lilia, Laurie, (such similar names) and especially Imelda who always made us both laugh. They made it easier for him to feel comfortable as he drove me to chemo every week and spent the long hours sitting and waiting for the infusion to finish. There are times when love is not passion, it is all shared responsibility, shared history, and being there no matter what.

Imelda was planning her wedding and now we were learning about Filipino weddings. She was taking a bit from the traditional ceremony and adding in a dash of Las Vegas glitz. How could I not love her? We had spent every Tuesday morning together for 15 weeks and now we were on the home stretch.

I was scheduled to finish week 18 on December 28 just after Christmas. Agustin had scheduled me for the post chemo PET and CT scans in January. I was scheduled for surgery in February and six weeks after surgery I would start back on bevacizumab and get an infusion every three weeks from April through November until I finished 12 more infusions. I had another full year of treatments ahead.

Cycle 6 was the last time I had the carboplatin infusion. And as I had come to expect, there were several bad days of vomiting that were difficult to control even with the medications. I knew how to get through it like an athlete pushing through pain. I did what I could to make myself comfortable, I tried to ignore it, I took the pills that Lilia prescribed, and I waited for it to pass. I was hoping that better days lay ahead.

The bottom line is this, in the 18 weeks, I probably had no more than 9 days when I experienced vomiting. I was miserable for a few days. The dry heaves felt painful in my stomach and my abdominal muscles. Nine days in 18 weeks, I didn't think was so bad. At the time it was unpleasant but tolerable, and I would do it again in a heartbeat. I know people are terrified of chemo, but chemo was a deal I would take any day.

Chapter 20: Feeling Older – Feeling Younger

I was looking forward to finishing chemo. I was counting down the cycles and the days. The chemo had brought the CA-125 down to the normal range. Yet, coming off chemo was surprisingly frightening just like starting chemo was frightening. I was afraid that without the chemo the cancer would regain ground and start growing back. What if there were a few cancer cells still left, what would keep them from starting to grow again?

It all came down to the unknown. Would that CA-125 start going up the very next visit? What was going to happen if it did? Would I start all over again on another drug? Would that work?

Chemo had become my security. I said again — cancer was my enemy and chemo was my friend — a PITA (pain in the ass) friend to be sure, but at that moment, still a protective friend. As I have talked with others who have been on chemo, I have found that most people experience this worry when chemo is finished. This is another and unexpected fear to add to all of the other fears in treating cancer, I was more afraid to stop the chemo than I was to initially start it.

Remarkably, a few weeks after my last chemo, I was already beginning to feel better. It happened faster than I expected. I felt a few years younger every week. My energy returned. I could think more clearly. In a few weeks I could eat most foods. The mouth sores cleared up; my stomach was settled. The neuropathy and achy feelings continued. But despite lingering effects, I felt like I was beginning to recognize my body again.

I was in the six-week break recovering from chemo and getting stronger to face surgery. My son David and his wife Ali came to visit from Rhode Island with their four-year old son Thomas and their two-year old son Trevor. My daughter Katherine and her husband Mike, not far away in Southern California and their three-year old Connor and one-year old Ryan were ready for fantasy.

They were all looking forward to visiting Disneyland, the Magic Kingdom, and perhaps some of that magic would rub off on me. So, despite my too-soon-after-chemo level of fitness. I didn't want to miss out. That was a real issue with chemo, I always felt like I was missing out on something and the fact is that I was.

I knew I would not last the day. The fatigue had not fully lifted and my brain was not yet completely clear. While everyone else was off early to be at the park when it opened, Jim and I slept late and didn't get there until 10 o'clock.

Coming off chemo, Disneyland is impossibly colorful, loud, and crowded. It was a shock to the illness-imposed quietude that had taken over my life. I knew I would not do whirling rides, or rides that went up and down or anything that spun me around or went fast. Even the Mad Hatter spinning teacups were out, as was the flying Dumbo ride, the Matterhorn, and everything else that would make a child squeal with excitement. Those rides would just make me dizzy and perhaps worse.

Disneyland used to be the land of Mickey, and I suppose it still owes a lot to *el raton,* however, for my young grandsons it was the land of Buzz Lightyear. Still, they were not prepared to see a six-foot tall costumed Buzz step out from behind a curtain, coming not from space, but from the tunnels and staging areas beneath their feet. Children imagine seeing the real Buzz as eighteen inches high, buzzing around overhead and saying "to infinity and beyond," which surely had no meaning to them. I have a clear image in my memory of four little boys looking baffled and maybe terrified by the enormous Buzz they encountered. And I remember laughing and saying to myself, "I am so lucky to be here."

Four hours later, we were at the far end of the park when I hit the wall of my endurance and was done. That is another reality of cancer treatment, you can be going along fine and then all of a sudden, the gas tank is empty and you just stop and cannot go any further. Four hours of walking, watching and laughing and I was ready to go home. Jim and I got on the train that encircles the park and took it back to the entrance where we got on a tram that took us to our car. I was asleep before we hit the freeway. But I was done with missing out. I wanted to get back to participating as soon as possible and this was a step forward that I was glad I did not skip.

A few weeks later, I went for the post chemo CT and PET scans. These would give the real answer about how well the chemo had worked and whether they showed cancer still remaining. The same nurse who had told me about her experience with breast cancer did the scans again. With her spiky short haircut, she assured me that soon my hair would come back. She congratulated me on finishing chemo. "I would just hug myself and repeat to myself, I will be well," she said again.

When I was in my office a few days later I received an email from Agustin telling me to call him about the scan results. Before I could even finish reading the email, enough to start worrying, he walked into my office and sat down.

"Your scans look completely normal," he said. "Dr. Henderson read them and compared them with the baseline scans. He was so excited that he called even before he wrote and sent the formal report. He said there is no evidence of disease on the scans."

I have pictures of those scans. My PET scans before chemo looked like a Christmas tree lit up every place the cancer had been. My scans after chemo looked like someone had pulled the plug and the lights were now out.

But questions remained. Instead of asking if the chemo would work, now I questioned whether or not there were tiny micro places where the cancer was still growing. Where might those places be? The chemo had gone all the way to my fingernails, to my brain, to every place that blood flowed all over my body. Nobody knew if there was a micro spot, though none were showing up on the scans. If it showed on the scan I would know it was there but if it did not show up, I would not know for sure that there was not a hidden micro spot. Ovarian cancer is one of those cancers that often responds well to initial therapy but very often recurs. The unanswerable questions continued and my worrying over them continued. At the same time, that I felt relieved and even triumphant, the uncertainty lingered.

Such good news after weeks of worry was so quietly delivered, no fireworks and no marching band. As it began to sink in I began to wonder. Is it possible that I could be well? I could not read Agustin's face well enough to know his feelings: pride, surprise, worry maybe a mixture.

How could I thank someone who got it right, who figured out what to do and helped me get through it? I was finished with the hard cytotoxic chemo. I still had more tests, surgery, and eight months of bevacizumab infusions planned. And then I would wait to see if the cancer came back. But right then, there was no evidence of disease (NED). The first phase of regaining my health had been successful. I had rounded first base, cleared the first jump, finished the first lap, and any other sports analogy I could think of, but I was still far from finished.

Later that day, walking down the hall, I saw Lilia my nurse practitioner. Her broad grin spread wide and her face lit up, "Did you hear? Did you talk with Agustin?"

"Yes, he told me. Amazing."

Chapter 21: Is the Decimal Misplaced?

Bevacizumab was one of the newer cancer drugs when I started treatment in 2010. It was being tested but had not been approved for ovarian cancer (and was not approved until 2014). Agustin warned me that since it was not approved by the FDA for my type of cancer, my insurance might not cover it and he was right. Initially the coverage was denied. I appealed but was denied a second time. Jim and I talked about paying for it out-of-pocket and not knowing the cost, we thought that would be possible. Agustin thought it would cost around $70,000 and that seemed a worthwhile way to spend some of my accumulated retirement savings. If it helped me get well then I might need to work extra years to replace those savings. And if it didn't, it would be money down the drain. We fully realized how fortunate we were to have that money and how many women would have had to say "no," they would not be able to commit to such an expense.

Medical bills are often delayed. The hospital bills the insurance first and then the patient, so the bills to the patient are especially slow. By the time the first bill came we were already in cycle four. The bill for the first infusion of just the bevacizumab alone was over $32,000. "This has got to be a mistake, they must have put the decimal in the wrong place," I said. "If it is really $32,000, 18 infusions would cost $576,000. This has to be wrong." It looked like a baggie of clear liquid. It just couldn't be that costly. Eighteen baggies could fit in our Coleman cooler. If it were going to cost $576,000, that would be more than the original cost of our house, our cars, and our children's college education combined.

I asked Agustin to appeal to the insurance company for me. He told me that the results of the clinical trial would be out in a month or so and he thought it would get approved for ovarian cancer. Once the clinical trial results came out, he would appeal. I left optimistic that it would get resolved, but I still thought there must be some mistake in the amount.

A few weeks later, I got a statement from the insurance company showing they paid $15,000 and the patient portion showed that I owed nothing. So, what happened to the other $17,000? Obviously, I was not going to ask.

A few weeks later, I got a bill for Cycle 2 – the bill was not the same amount but again it was for over $32,000 to me, the patient. "This is nuts," I thought.

"Just put that bill in the drawer and forget about it," said one of my nurses.

This made me laugh, but I also didn't know how to deal with it and I just hoped the insurance company would pay it again. But I also had fear that they would decide they had erroneously paid for the first infusion and might reverse that. I certainly was not going to call them and say "hey, you paid for the first one – why not the second?" Although I could not forget about it, I decided to finish chemo and then figure it out; I had enough on my mind. So, in violation of everything I learned from my accountant father, the bills went in the drawer in my desk though they were never hidden from my book-balancing brain. Instead of paying them, I just hoped.

Pretty soon I got a statement saying Cycle 2 was paid also.

"I guess Agustin got it straightened out," I thought. He must have persuaded them to cover it and that the cost was wrong and that is why they paid half the amount.

The next time I saw him I thanked him for appealing and getting it covered by insurance. "I never appealed," he said, "I was waiting for the final trial data."

"Well, they paid it," I said, "something must have changed their mind." He didn't know and I didn't know – and I never got a letter explaining.

This continued over the 18 infusions. I would irregularly get bills that were paid while others were not paid, and I had no idea what was happening.

I couldn't understand why this one drug cost so much, or how to make sure the insurance company paid it all. Further, while I was almost done with the 6 infusions of bevacizumab before surgery, I only had bills for three; and there were 12 more infusions planned after surgery. I began to wonder if I should stop this drug. What if the insurance didn't keep paying and I had to pay it all and it might not even work? But what if I stopped this drug and what if I cut my chances of surviving because I discontinued it? Eventually the other bills came and sometimes follow-up bills and then I got statements saying payment was denied and then got another statement saying it was paid. In the end the insurance company paid about half of what the hospital billed, which was still an outrageous amount, and the balance seemed to vanish into thin air. I never knew or got any communication that explained this chaotic billing situation or explained why the insurance company paid these bills after denying payment. What changed their mind about paying? But I do wonder if it was because I was being treated in a research center. Sometimes I wonder if a kindly claims clerk just decided to pay it all. Who knows? Once the bills were paid, I chose never to ask.

Medical billing makes no sense. Insurance companies get billed by the hospitals for outrageous amounts; they pay a portion of it and the rest – who knows what happens to it? It's like going to a restaurant, getting charged four times what it should be, then saying you will only pay a portion of it and everyone says "fine." What business operates like this? The difference here is that both the hospital and the insurance company are in on the game. Hospitals know they will only get a portion of what they bill so they begin by inflating the bill never expecting to get paid this inflated amount. When they do get paid, they either say "fine" or they try to collect more from the patient. There are agreements between insurance companies and hospitals so that hospitals get the amount they need in order to function and survive.

Patients don't know what the game is. Very ill patients get outrageous bills that they know they cannot pay at a time when they are already in a state of extreme stress from their disease and treatment. Patients may withdraw from treatment because they cannot handle the bills, and they don't want this expense to be a burden on their families. Medical bills are also a major cause of personal bankruptcy and eventually this can lead to homelessness. How many women don't get optimal care because of unexpected medical bills? I might not have continued with this drug after surgery if the bills had not been paid. If this drug in combination with the other chemo was the key to my survival, then without it, I might not have survived. How often is lifesaving treatment denied by insurance companies? How many people go bankrupt due to these inflated bills? How many forgo treatment to avoid these bills? And what should these drugs really cost?

It is not the purpose of this book to critique the pharmaceutical industry. However, a simple internet search of the CEOs of pharmaceutical companies gives information on the staggering compensation (salary, bonuses, and stock) received by these individuals. The New York Times also publishes an annual report on CEO salaries for the largest companies in the United States. The compensation often exceeds $20 million per year for pharmaceutical company CEOs. To date, there is virtually no control over CEO salaries or over pharmaceutical costs in the US.

PART III: AND THEN SURGERY

Chapter 22: Surgery Knocked me Down

Surgery was planned for mid-February. I had six weeks to get my strength back and take a breather after the months of chemotherapy.

My surgeon, Laila, was a friend, yet the thought of having parts of my body removed and examined under a microscope was unnerving, even though those parts were making me sick and I knew they needed to go. I wanted them out but I didn't want to have surgery. This is like being nine months pregnant and not wanting to go through labor. It's just not possible. It doesn't work that way. The only way forward was through the surgery door.

A week before surgery I had my pre-operative visit to check for heart function and to sign papers. I was given a package that contained the disinfecting towels to use before surgery. This pre-surgical preparation was required to avoid infections. The day before surgery, bed sheets had to be washed, I had to shower and wash carefully with soap, and after that Jim had to help me wipe each quadrant of my body with a separate one of the disinfecting towels that left me feeling slightly sticky. Similarly, in the morning I needed to be careful to not contaminate myself in any way. Everything my skin touched was clean. I kept telling myself to "stay calm", this would be over soon and then I could get back to "normal" —"new normal."

Jim and I got to the lobby of the Norris Cancer Hospital early the next morning. There were patients waiting to be called for surgery, some with a spouse, some with a son or daughter, and some with an entire family. When my name was called, Jim and I went up the elevator to the surgical floor. I was assigned to a pre-surgical bed with a curtain separating me from the next bed and the next person waiting for surgery. I changed into the hospital gown and got into the bed to wait.

A young resident came to the foot of my bed holding a clipboard. She introduced herself as a doctor. A new doctor I thought. She needed to get my consent for surgery. She confirmed my name and date of birth. And then she read "sixty-two-year-old woman with Stage IV ovarian cancer consenting to total removal of ovaries, fallopian tubes, and uterus" and on it went – "please sign here to consent to surgery."

"Yes, I understand" I said several times, "I understand." I wanted to say, I had Stage IV cancer five months ago, but now I don't – now they can't find anything on the scans, so it is not stage IV anymore. I wanted to shake that label but I was stuck with it. I will always be classified as Stage IV. I felt like a felon who served my time but would always be called a felon. "Give it a rest," I thought. "Stop saying that." But of course, she didn't.

And then the anesthesia resident came to my bedside and I went through the whole thing again. She confirmed my name and birthdate. "Sixty-two-year-old women with Stage IV ovarian cancer consenting to total removal of ovaries, fallopian tubes, and uterus, please sign here to consent to anesthesia."

I felt like I was trying to hold onto my version of reality and all of the residents were treating me like I had not just gone through 18 weeks of chemo and now had clear scans. They might think I would be filled with cancer, when they opened me up, but I knew that was not true. If they found any, it would have to be small because it did not show up on the scans.

I could see other patients being wheeled through the doors to the operating suites and I was still waiting. "Let's get on with this," I said. Jim said, "I'm sure it will be soon. Just hang on."

Laila showed up and told me that there was a slight delay. They were one staff short and a replacement was on the way. It will be soon she said and then left to get ready. I was the only one left in the pre-operative area.

A half hour later, an anesthesia nurse said the team was ready. She gave me a shot and she started to push my bed toward the two swinging doors that led to the hallway and then to the surgical suites. We went through the swinging doors, I looked up and saw what I assume were young physicians and nurses on each side of my bed as I was pushed through and that was the last thing I remembered until I woke up in the recovery room.

A nurse was shouting at me "Jean, wake up." She pulled over another nurse. "What is that?" she said and her agitation was obvious.

It slowly dawned on me that I was in recovery and that surgery was over. I was too groggy to focus or even formulate a question and I fell back to sleep.

Again, "Jean, wake up!"

I tried to look around. "What time is it?" I asked. It seemed late. Did she hear me? Did any sound come out?

"We're waiting for a bed in the ICU," she said.

Was that the plan? I didn't remember that.

I slept and waited a while longer and then my bed was pushed out of recovery and I was looking at the ceiling lights as I went down long hallways on my way to the ICU. Basements of hospitals are dreary places and are the expressway for patients being transferred around the hospital. The aide pushing my bed greeted others who were pushing other patients in the opposite direction. It was clear there was an entire social network among the transport aides in the basement and I, as a patient, was extraneous to the ongoing greeting and waving only occasionally asked if I was OK, which I was despite feeling helpless and foggy brained.

When I got to the ICU, I was turned over to the ICU nurse in a bay with lots of machines. "Look at this," the recovery nurse was saying to the ICU nurse as she showed her readouts from what I assumed was a heart monitoring machine. I heard her say, "What is this? I have not seen this before." They continued to look at machines and I continued to be out of the loop. I still did not know what all of the agitation was about.

"What's wrong?" I asked. "Your heart beat is irregular," she said "we need to monitor you."

"My heart? I don't have heart problems." So now I had gone from ovary problems to heart problems?

Jim showed up at last. I immediately felt safer. "What time is it?"

"It's after seven" he said. "How are you feeling?"

"OK. Really, it has been 12 hours?"

And then the resident showed up. It was her job to check on me. "Dr. Muderspach checked on you in recovery. She will be back in the morning." I didn't remember seeing her.

"You have bigeminy," she said. This is a term I didn't know and asked her to explain.

"You heart is irregular; it is supposed to go thump thump thump thump thump – very regular. Yours is going thump thump pause, thump thump pause, thump thump." I was unaware of the unusual heart beat and I began taking my pulse to see if I could feel it in my postsurgical brain fog and I felt nothing — no pulse at all. I probably was not up to taking my own pulse, but it did feel unnerving. Lingering logic told me I must have a pulse since I was still alive and the heart monitor machine was still beeping and showing charts of a beating heart.

"Why is it doing that? Is this dangerous? Will it go back to normal?"

The answers were: "Don't know. Don't know. Don't know."

I decided I would ask Laila in the morning, but for right now, I just needed to try to start recovering. Maybe in the morning the anesthesia would wear off and everything would go back to normal.

In the morning after a sleepless night filled with beeping and lights, people walking by and blood draws, Laila came by to check on me. She talked with the ICU doctor who advised against bringing in a cardiologist, he wanted to give my body time to fix itself. Laila trusted him and I trusted her. I believed my body would settle.

"When can I go home?"

"You need to be able to eat, walk, urinate and have a bowel movement, and we need to be sure this heart issue is not a problem."

With that as the goal, I asked my nurse to help me walk down the hallway, and off we went, past the other ICU bays as we slowly dragged the various machines that were monitoring me. We made it to the end of the hall and then back to the chair in my ICU cubicle. Walking was painful and I was exhausted.

A little while later the ICU doctor, a small quiet man who seemed unimpressed with my heart problems, and a bunch of junior doctors came in to talk to me. "How are you feeling?" he asked.

"Fine," I said – the habit of trying to be pleasant and agreeable made this answer seem almost comical. I had been raised by my Irish mother to avoid complaining and to be polite, especially to doctors who were trying to help me. But really how was I feeling? Well, I was in pain, I couldn't even comfortably walk down the hall, I was hungry, and more than anything I wanted to go home and sleep. I am sure I did not look very fine in my hospital gown with my bald head and sitting hunched over to ease my belly pain. That word "fine" covers a lot of territory. But that and all of the machines seemed to satisfy the ICU doctor and he moved on like a trail guide with the newbie doctors. At some level though, I was grateful to him. He didn't call in more specialists and further complicate the matter and I continued to trust my body to settle down.

At the end of the day, I was moved to a room on a regular floor. I went from being completely in the center of action in the ICU to the last room at the end of the hall, furthest from the nursing station. I appreciated the quiet end of the hall but almost felt forgotten and I began to wonder if anyone would show up if I needed help. The windows looked out toward the San Gabriel Mountains, towards my home, where I was yearning to go as soon as possible.

When Jim showed up on Saturday morning I was anxious to get moving. "You need to help me walk down the hall — I want to go home tomorrow so I need to get walking." Off we went with me walking slowly and stooped over, in a robe, achy and holding onto the hall railings and with Jim steadying me. Right away I ran into a colleague, an oncologist, who had her office right around the corner from mine. She had a great wardrobe and true to form she was in a beautiful suit and stiletto heels. This was just what I didn't want — to see anyone I knew in this condition. She looked surprised to see me and I felt embarrassed to see her. "Yes, I had surgery Thursday. Yes, Laila is my surgeon. This is my husband, Jim. I want to go home tomorrow so I need to take a walk. See you later." I felt like adding "alligator" which was a stupid thing that popped into my mind from childhood. We moved on. "Keep walking and do what you need to do I coached myself." "In a while crocodile."

When Laila came by the next morning, my thoughts were clear enough to ask questions and remember the answers. "I didn't find any cancer," she said. "We had the original scans and we took tissue from those areas where it was before. We had a pathologist in the operating room and the tissue was checked as we went along. We didn't find any remaining cancer. All of the tissue will be sent to the pathology lab and they will section it and then we will know for sure. It went well but it took a long time. It's as good an outcome as I have ever seen."

I was smiling and tearing up at the same time.

"I'm walking, eating, urinating and passing gas – is that good enough – can I go home?"

"Yes, we will monitor you for a few more hours but you can go home this afternoon."

The human body is both fragile and resilient. After 18 weeks of chemo, major surgery and a two-night hospital stay, I recovered more quickly than I thought possible.

In my life before cancer, I never expected to need major surgery. I had always regarded my body as healthy and expected it to stay intact my entire life. Yet it was completely clear that surgery was essential despite my clear scans and normal marker counts. But how would it feel afterwards I wondered? Would there be a feeling of emptiness where once vital organs dwelled?

I have talked with women who described their surgery as being "gutted." If there ever was a horrible term, that has got to be it. It is formally called "debulking" which is only slightly better sounding. If the cancer has spread to other organs, the intestines or the colon then those may need to be resected which means the cancerous part is cut out and the colon reconnected. But in a few cases the surgery is even more extensive and a colostomy is performed which means that the intestine exits to the outside on the abdomen and the woman then needs to wear a colostomy bag to collect feces that can no longer exit through the rectum. Sometimes these colostomies can be reversed and sometimes they cannot. Susan Gubar a respected feminist professor of literature, has described her difficult life living with this extensive surgery in her book *"Memoir of a Debulked Woman."* Yes, in those cases, I can understand why women feel "gutted."

My reality was that I felt no different, no grieving for the lost body parts and no feeling of emptiness. The incisions were painful but because Laila had performed robotic surgery, the five incisions about one inch long each around my waist line were small and I recovered fast. Now ten years later the incision scars are not even noticeable.

I thought my stomach would be suddenly flat and I would lose several pounds. But wrong again, neither of these good results occurred either. Of course, this makes sense since the uterus and ovaries together weigh less than a quarter of a pound.

I put myself on a walking plan starting in the house, then up and down the stairs to the second floor, then back and forth in the yard, and 10 days after surgery Jim and I went to a level street and I was able to walk a mile. This was not an energetic mile and by the end I was tired and sore; but it was a determined mile and it was a start. Little by little my energy returned. And it led me to my belief that "walking is medicine."

PART IV: COMING TO TERMS WITH MY LIFE WITH CANCER

Chapter 23: Illness and Piety with a Side of Prayer

Cancer caused a reckoning. It caused me to examine and challenge myself. It caused me to look back and evaluate how I had lived my life, my values and beliefs, my faith, my determination to deal with the threat and demands of treatment, my relationships, and my thoughts on dying. These struggles went on in my mind, and at times led to panic, meditative acceptance, resilience, and often to a confusing mix of all of these.

The link between religious beliefs and illness is fraught with confusion. Historically and even recently, there are pious souls who consider those afflicted with various illnesses as sinful and the illness itself demonstrating God's judgment. In ancient times it was leprosy, in our time it was AIDS that evoked these responses. There are those who consider illnesses to be sent from God, or within God's control, or ignored by God. Some see illness as a means to test faith itself. They look at the story of Job and wonder if they too are being tested. They may see a religious meaning in suffering. After all, the scripture says that God is omnipotent and omniscient, all powerful and all knowing, and if that is true then where does that lead? Is God letting this happen, ignoring it, or just does not care? How can this be reconciled?

When I was diagnosed, I had no formulaic explanations to ease my acceptance. I did not believe I was being punished like the Egyptians who suffered plagues because they would not let the children of Israel free, nor did I believe that God was testing me like Job in the Old Testament. And if everything happens for a reason as some believe, the reason was certainly not clear to me. But I knew more about what I did not believe than what I did believe. For me the gulf between this illness and faith was irreconcilable. They seemed to be two separate tracks, not intersecting or related and both going in directions that pointed only to loss and confusion.

My husband, Jim, was raised in a conservative Christian family originally gathered into a small denomination called Brethren. Smoking, drinking, card-playing, gambling, movies, and dancing – both damaging and innocent pastimes were avoided. The Brethren believed, "Live simply that others may simply live." And despite financial and other successes, for the most part, they adhered to the modest and quiet lifestyle of their faith.

When his father died suddenly of a heart attack at age 43, when Jim was 12 and his brother 16 and sister 9, the explanations to those children were enough to fracture anyone's belief in a just or kind God. "God loved your father so much that he wanted him to be with Him." "He is with God and he is watching over you." "Everything happens for a reason; faith will make that reason clear." "Do not be sad, he is in a better place, with God." "The angels are not crying." What child would not resent this God? And yet the explanations, however nonsensical and even harmful, persisted and questioning was stifled. And 10 years later, when his brother was diagnosed with Hodgkin lymphoma at age 26, the explanations had not changed and they still did not work.

Life's greatest challenges bring beliefs and coping mechanisms to a collision course. While belief in God may be a comfort at one level, at another level it raises questions about the love of God and the justice and fairness of God, questions that are unanswerable and age old. "Why do bad things happen to good people?" "Why did God let this happen?" And these questions are asked in response to individual suffering but also for the shared suffering of millions due to genocide, hunger, poverty, war and so much more. We all persist in asking. But the only answers I have found exist in the uncontrollable natural world of diseases and natural disasters or in the venality and selfishness of leaders who seek money, land, and power and forget the poor and the ill. The natural or the man made – these are the common sources of suffering.

Faith is a troublesome thing for me. Biblical teachings provide guidance for my life and my understanding of right and wrong, but that is the simple part. It is faith in a higher being or spirit, spiritual faith that is the problem. There are years when the existence of God seems close and easier to believe – and there are years when the existence of God seems like a delusional explanation for both the good and bad things that happen in life. And I take comfort in reading that Mother Teresa, a devout follower if ever there was one, experienced distance and even abandonment in her belief, yet she continued her justice and healing ministry.

And yet I prayed.

My friend Sheila told me that when she was first diagnosed with HIV, she "hit her knees." And I hit my knees as well. The saying goes that, " there are no atheists in a foxhole." When someone is shooting at you and you have only a foxhole to protect you, you get on your knees and pray. Because that is the only thing you can do that brings comfort. This makes sense for cancer also.

I was uncertain if God would hear my prayers and more than that, I was uncertain about what I thought or believed about God and especially about the control God might have on my cancer. And yet when I was diagnosed, it was this distant and perhaps unhearing God that I prayed to. Over and over again "*let the chemo work, kill the cancer, let me be well, let me see my grandchildren grow up, let me live, can't you see I have more to give?, can't you see it would be a better thing for me to live and contribute to a better world than to die now?, let me live, let the chemo work, I will never complain again,* " and so on and so on and over and over again. I was bargaining with God, trying to convince myself that my arguments were persuasive. I was certain I had good works in front of me, more research and teaching and certainly more acts of generosity. It seemed like such a waste. But I suspect everyone feels that way.

And not only did I pray, I asked for the prayers of others.

There was one person that I was certain I wanted to pray for me, who I thought might have the ear of God. My husband's Aunt Betty was for me the image of constant and simple faith, lived out every day in her kind and generous life consistent with her Christian beliefs. By the time I developed cancer she was nearly ninety years old, and she had difficulty speaking even though her thoughts were clear. It felt odd and even superstitious to ask, and yet I knew that if she was praying for me I would somehow feel just a bit safer.

And then somehow I got a thought that if 100 people prayed for me, I would be well. Why 100? Where did this thought even come from?

I found it uplifting to know that because my friends came from many religious traditions, the prayers were diverse and maybe my bases were covered. My friend Alexandra went to temple on Rosh Hashanah and entered my name in the Book of Life. My friend Lourdes arranged for priests to pray for me at the Grotto of Lourdes in France. She gave me a card with the exact days that I was prayed for at this site, so holy in her faith. I put myself on the prayer list at church. A friend put me on an international prayer network. People I didn't even know were praying for me. I had prayers in English and in Spanish, which was good since I am sure God is at least bilingual.

Jim's family prayed for me from their evangelical perspective. My Muslim friends prayed for me also and in that tradition, believers pray five times a day, which seems like a lot, but maybe they are short – I don't really know. Jim and I prayed together at night holding each other in bed. Even my good friends who declared themselves atheists said they were offering good thoughts, sending messages to the universe in some way that they were uncomfortable calling a prayer but I am not sure what else to call it. Some of these friends crossed their fingers, as though that makes more sense to them than praying. In some mysterious way knowing that people were praying for me added to my sense of security and strengthened me.

A friend came to visit me while I was having a chemo infusion and later sent me an email that I vacillated between marveling at and dismissing – finally deciding to add it to my reception of strengthening prayers. Her note said:

> *"When I walked into the room you had a white robe on, the sheets were white, and there seemed to be a white glow in the room. I was transfixed as I got closer to you because it was as though there was this white light glowing all around your head. I didn't say anything about it to you at the moment, because I didn't understand it, but it caused a profound impression in me. On my ride home I called my mom and I told her what I had seen. She said it had been revealed to me that you would be healed, because that was your aura; and it was proof you were being cleansed by the pureness of your heart. "*

I don't know about the pureness of my heart, although I do try. I did not see the white glow so maybe it was her pure heart since she was the one who saw it and I can absolutely vouch for her good heart and her faith is beyond mine. Her note did cause me to wonder at the things that are beyond our understanding.

My church is involved in causes of homelessness, health care for the poor, AIDS care, anti-racism, immigration, foster children, environmental protection, civil rights, gun control, gay rights, gender equality, and a host of other causes often associated with liberal positions. Liberal is from the French for "liberty" I might add, and hence for me a very positive and American characteristic.

My church has liturgical traditions from the Book of Common Prayer. Every Sunday, immediately after communion, those wishing prayers for healing can kneel and receive personal prayers from the clergy. It is not exactly the mystical "laying on of hands," even though hands are laid on the head or shoulder of those kneeling. A visiting priest who had the look of a bearded short Santa Claus, after I told him my diagnosis, wrapped his hands around my head and prayed such a long and personal prayer for healing that when he was finished my tears, that had been held back all week long, were released, and it felt like somehow God must have heard him.

Every Wednesday a much smaller service was held for healing and about 20 people gathered. That service was my chance to lay my hands on others and pray for them. And it was their chance to pray for me. There were people with cancer, with depression, with immune problems and with heart problems – there were people anticipating surgery and some recovering from surgery. And there were those who were helping their family members go through hard times as well. These services are an expression of reliance on God and supplication when nothing seems to be clear or even possible to control. They were a gathering of a supportive community bonded by individual trials.

Zelda, a tall African American priest with a big smile and a warm hug, was especially devoted to pastoral care and this healing ministry. Her prayers and presence were a sustaining force for me. She prayed for me on many Wednesdays and when I went into remission we prayed a prayer of thanks together. Several years later she developed breast cancer and though many prayed for her she did not survive. If survival were all about how many were praying for her, she would still be alive today.

But I did not appreciate all prayers. Too often I heard the well-intentioned "I'm praying for you" not as a genuine response but as an avoidance – it ended conversation and put the focus on the actions of the other person. What I heard was not the pious assurance of prayers but the avoidance of discussion. I heard this: "I don't want to talk about this with you but I want you to think I am a caring person – so I will tell you I am praying for you." At one point I wrote an angry rant about these prayers.

Does prayer really matter?
I think so, but kindness matters more.
Don't say you pray for me
    if you never show up.
Don't say you care
    if you don't call.
Don't tell me of your piety
    if you don't visit.
Are your prayers for yourself ?
Do they convince you of your own goodness?

Does God even listen if that is so?
I don't think so.
Pray for yourself then –
pray that you get a heart capable of more –
a heart that makes you move from your pew and
lift your head from your Bible and
makes you reach out of your own righteousness
and
help someone else.
In the end, if you pray and
don't show up –
it just makes me angry and
right now
that is the last thing I need.

When I went into remission, these same people were only too happy to credit their own prayers – their prayers were answered. If only such power were in their prayers. "Get real," I want to say to them, but instead I say "thank you." Because what kind of person would not graciously accept prayers - and besides – who knows? But I do feel that other peoples fear of cancer led to some, even those professing piety to abandon me. I had to contend with this, until I survived, and then they wanted to hear all about it.

Prayer does not stand alone. In the absence of loving support, it is not worth much. But in that moment of loving support, understanding, and the absence of trite explanations – it is a powerful means of strengthening the wanderings of the frightened mind that invariably surround the cancer diagnosis. Does prayer cure cancer? I think not. Does God hear prayers? I hope so. Did prayer help me live through the experience? Yes, I believe it did. And that is enough.

Chapter 24: Wit, John Donne, Dylan Thomas, Kubler-Ross, and Me

One of my junior colleagues who I had known for many years, brought me a DVD one day after I had just finished chemo. The title was *Wit* and it was starring the wonderful British actress Emma Thompson. I knew of this title as a Broadway play about an ill woman. But I had paid it little attention.

"It's about ovarian cancer," she said. "I thought you might like to watch it." I don't know what possessed her to lend me this film. I am sure she was well meaning.

But, before I go on, let me just say, don't ever give this film to anyone who has just been diagnosed or is undergoing treatment for ovarian cancer and for sure don't take that person to a public place to see this play unless you are prepared to see a full avalanche of grief poured out in the seat next to you complete with sobbing and shaking and leaving in a mess of tissues and stares.

Margaret Edson wrote this play about ovarian cancer in 1991. After finishing her studies in Renaissance history, she found herself employed selling hotdogs, bartending, and working as an assistant in an AIDS and cancer hospital. *Wit* is the story of an arrogant and unlikeable English professor, Vivian Bearing, who is an expert on the sonnets of John Donne, a poet and clergyman in the time of Queen Elizabeth I. Edson sent the play to 60 theaters and it was rejected, the topic after all is about dying. It was finally accepted at one theater and despite critical success, it took several years before it made its way to theaters in New York City and then it won the Pulitzer Prize for Drama in 1999, and an Emmy for the film version in 2001. Edson then became an elementary school teacher and never wrote another play.

In the play, Bearing is diagnosed with Stage IV ovarian cancer and is treated with chemotherapy. She wants to show she can take all of the chemo, full dose, no breaks and she takes some pride in that tenacity. And here I see a similarity to myself. But unlike me, she becomes sicker and weaker and in pain.

She reflects on her life's work and on a particular sonnet by John Donne, called Holy Sonnet 10 but usually referred to as *Death be not Proud.*

Death be not proud, though some have called thee
Mighty and dreadful, for thou art not so;
For those whom thou think'st thou dost overthrow
Die not, poor Death, nor yet canst thou kill me.......

One short sleep past, we wake eternally
And death shall be no more; Death thou shalt die

As a clergyman, Donne believed that death is a temporary state that it is quickly followed by resurrection, life after death and eternal life. Not surprising, this poem is often read at funerals.

Vivian tenaciously holds onto her life undergoing difficult and experimental treatments that do not help her. In the play, only one nurse provides her comfort as she struggles with her illness and treatment, but the physicians and in fact the entire hospital system are cold and uncaring. My experience was different. Everywhere I turned I was cared for with kindness from phlebotomists, nurses, physicians, and radiology technicians. And at some level the play seems like an unfair indictment. But Vivian herself had always been cold and uncaring to her students and it seems she received as she had given.

As she is dying, only her academic mentor visits her. She asks if Vivian would like to hear the Donne poem. But Vivian chooses to hear the children's story, *The Runaway Bunny,* about the unconditional love of a parent who will find and protect her child wherever her child might run or hide. The sonnet mocks death as though it was a person perhaps the grim reaper. It challenges the struggle and finality of death. This was not comforting to Vivian and perhaps it did not speak truth as she dealt with her own suffering and impending death. The simplicity of a children's story about love comforted her.

I imagine that Margaret Edson studied John Donne as a Renaissance major. Perhaps she had a professor like Vivian Bearing. I imagine that working in a cancer and AIDS ward brought her to see the reality of how difficult dying and death can be. Perhaps she met a woman dying of ovarian cancer, maybe someone like Vivian. Maybe she was haunted by that person and in writing *Wit,* she told that woman's story.

But at some level I am angry at Margaret Edson. She wrote a play that left little hope for women with ovarian cancer. She portrayed those who make their life work caring for such patients and researching ways to improve treatments as cold and unconcerned with their patients' suffering. And in the end the message is dire. What woman who has seen this play or the movie version would be able to face this disease and treatment with confidence?

Centuries later Dylan Thomas, a Welsh poet, wrote another famous poem about dying, *Do Not go Gentle Into that Good Night.*

> *"Do not go gentle into that good night,*
> *Old age should burn and rave at close of day,*
> *Rage, rage against the dying of the light."*

It is also read at funerals, it has inspired paintings and orchestral works, and it has served many as a model of how to face death.

> *"Rage Rage against the dying"*

Thomas is said to have written it observing the aging of his own father who died five years later in 1952. Thomas himself died the following year in November 1953 – the death of a young alcoholic at age 39.

Did he rage? I wonder. He drank himself into a coma and died. But somehow I doubt that he raged — rather he slipped as if falling down through slippery dust with his mind only partially understanding that he was killing himself in a semiconscious way. In a stumbling stupor, not aware of his own actions or able to form coherent thoughts, neither raging nor welcoming but rather willing himself into the state where he was capable of neither. While he asked his father to rage, he likely slowly allowed his brain to shut down and his breathing to stop quietly in the end.

Rage?

No

Gentle?

Not that either.

These poems are perhaps the most famous poems about how to face death. And why is that? What do we see or want to see in these poems?

These two poems are bookends of ways to articulate and think about death. One is based on belief in an afterlife and hence avoiding the reality of dying by believing it is only temporary. While Donne may offer peace that death is followed by resurrection, nobody can know for sure that it is or is not true. The peace that is given may be a lie and useful only in that it may comfort the dying person. The other is agnostic about an afterlife but raging to preserve the earthly life and angry that it will, in all cases, end. But they are similar as well. At some level, they both seem to believe that death can be conquered. Donne in his way is trying to take the power of death away by stating that it is simply not real or final, it is an illusion that the living see but the dead are alive in another state. Thomas faces the reality of death with rage and fear believing that in raging, strength-of-will can forestall dying. The finality of death is resisted with any force of spirit possible, and in so doing, death can be pushed back.

Yet I wonder under what circumstances these poems might speak truth. Certainly, there are times when fighting for life means that life will be extended. Certainly, also there are times when fighting for life just means that the dying becomes torturous and extended and futile and without peace of any sort. And if the raging fails, is it because there was a weak will to live? Is the person who dies at fault? And from Donne's perspective, do those who rage demonstrate a lack of faith and are at fault for that?

I wrestled with these questions as I reflected on my mortality and the finality of life and the limitations of life. Where is the fine line? Where is the noble path? How do we walk the tightrope as we approach death? Can we really take away the power and the finality by believing in an afterlife? Can we forestall it by raging? Which of these is comforting? I learned to hold both thoughts in my mind simultaneously, the determination and effort to live and the understanding that life does end and at some time that end must be accepted. But the confusion of cancer is knowing when each of these is the right path and when determination may need to yield to the power and certainty of death.

There is work to be done at the end of life. One thing about cancer is that it often allows that long preparation period. One of my doctors said there were worse ways to die. Sudden death does not allow the reconciliation that a cancer death usually allows. Cancer allows that time to consider, make peace, say what is often held back, understand the limitation of the human body, understand that a disease may be too unrelenting, understand that to go peacefully is a gift to the dying and to those who look on in grief. Raging does not give that peace.

The famous psychiatrist Dr. Elisabeth Kubler-Ross formalized the process of dying in her book *On Death and Dying.* Her work with dying patients led her to identify five phases of dying: denial, anger, bargaining, depression, and acceptance. She believed that those dying rotate through these stages in a somewhat orderly fashion. But it may be that only those who had Kubler-Ross at their bedside counseling them, were able to be so orderly about their impending death.

I recognize these stages but I believe they are more like a whirlwind of emotion cycling back and forth like a roulette wheel. The emotions may bounce through these stages and hopefully finally end in the acceptance slot.

Dylan Thomas was perhaps, at least in terms of his father's death, stuck in the anger and rage emotion. Donne seemed to deny all of the stages and what may appear to have been acceptance might have been bargaining or denial.

What does it mean to die well? What is a good death? It certainly cannot mean raging. It cannot mean welcoming death either. It is a wrenching away. It must mean grief and communal loss. Death is a loss to all and that is why we grieve.

Donne also wrote the poem *For Whom the Bell Tolls.*

> *Each man's death diminishes me,*
> *For I am involved in mankind.*
> *Therefore, send not to know*
> *For whom the bell tolls,*
> *It tolls for thee.*

And this poem speaks to me. It is about loss to the community. It is about being ripped away. The family and friends grieve and the loss can ripple beyond that circle. The impact on the family, the children left behind, the spouse now alone, the plans interrupted, all of these create the vacuum where once that person may have held so much together. The family is weaker and the community is weaker. But hopefully those people will learn to accept, will make new plans, will create new bonds and will welcome the continuing days. But yet the bell will toll for each of us and part of our job must be the easing of pain for the community.

The wrenching away is very different for the dying person. The dying person loses everyone, as well as the sun on a warm beach, the moon reflecting off the water, the stars on the desert, the oak trees dropping acorns, the dogs begging for cheese, Beethoven and the Beatles, pot roast and pralines. The person who is dying is not traveling the path of enduring a loss and then moving on. The dying person loses everything and does not move on, and that realization is terrifying, unless Donne is right, and I hope he is. But even if he is, does this belief make the process of dying and the uncertainty and terror easier to bear? For some, I suspect it does. But I think this is rare. The tenacity to hold onto life, to see a tomorrow, is a strong pull and not easily nullified by spiritual beliefs. That capitulation to death may only occur when it is clear that there is no other choice and any possibility for comfort may only exist in the spiritual.

Chapter 25: How Do We Learn How to Die?

My mother was an Irish immigrant; on a ship at 6-months old, she passed the Statue of Liberty on her way to Ellis Island. Her parents left Belfast with my mother, her 2-year-old brother and her 4-year-old sister and crossed the Atlantic to begin their lives in the promised land, America, or in their case, Newark, New Jersey. The year was 1919, the year that Ireland after decades of internal fighting was separated into the North and South largely divided on the basis of allegiance or hostility to England that had been going on for generations. The truth is, she told me, "All of the Irish, Protestant and Catholic, were as poor as church mice."

Enough of her extended family had immigrated to America and Canada that they could continue their clannish ways. Their accents were thick, and as a child I would sometimes be unable to understand my Irish grandparents. My mother laughed at my confusion as she put on a strong Irish accent and said "shurin the're speekin English, da ya na unerstan em?" My Irish grandparents were handsome people, a gift they passed on to their three children. My mother had a broad smile and green eyes. Her hair was thick and auburn and in my growing up years I thought she looked like the 1950's actress, Maureen O'Hara, only spoiled by gaining weight and fighting for years to lose it.

My mother was diagnosed with multiple myeloma at age 66 although the symptoms were there for several years before. Despite numerous doctor visits for mounting infections that should have signaled a diminished immune system, she was not diagnosed until she and my father (ever the accountant) went to a free community blood screening for seniors, and got a call that things were not right with her.

Multiple myeloma is a cancer of the blood plasma cells, the ones that make antibodies. These cancerous cells not only fail at their job of fighting infection, they also multiply in excess in the bone marrow to the point that they can fracture bones from the inside and can cause terrible bone pain. A few years after her diagnosis and on continual chemo she fell and broke both of her legs which kept her in a wheel chair or in bed the remainder of her life. The fractures were most likely caused by the cancer cells pushing on the bone from within and these fractures caused her fall.

The remainder of her life was riven by pain, immobility and increasing weight loss until she was only a fraction of the beautiful, auburn-haired woman with the Maureen O'Hara good looks and the broad smile.

Even then she would call friends when she heard they were ill. "I'm sorry I can't visit but tell me how you are," she would say, and then she and her friend would talk and laugh and comfort each other. It was the best she could accomplish of her lifetime habit of visiting or helping sick family or friends, and, despite her own illness, to not do this would have been a point of shame for her.

As we sat with her in the last weeks of her life, there was little more than skin covering her bones at the end and I wished for my robust mother of my childhood. She would not eat and soon she could not speak. We had a round the clock vigil sitting with her as she became comatose, maintaining her on injectable morphine because she could no longer take the oral pain pills. Her skin became hot to the touch and I feared it would come off in my hands as we turned her to prevent bed sores. For the days leading to her death at the very end of her life, I knew that for her, not only was the end near, but it needed to happen. Despite that, she lingered beyond the days the hospice nurses expected and those final days were the nightmare of cancer. We cared for her in the bedroom and in the bed that I had as a child. She died in my bed during my brother's vigil, and he woke us to say she was gone.

I can remember the breath going out of me as I looked at her. The relief at the end mixed with the grief that brought a choking sob from my core that had been held at bay for weeks and maybe longer. I can remember needing to get outside, to walk, to feel the air, to look around and see life in the trees, to feel the sun, and to experience life in my own body as I walked down the road to the small brook at the end where I had spent so many hours in my childhood catching frogs and turtles and salamanders.

People who say they are not afraid of dying have never seen a death like that. They have never seen that pain and wasting and daily loss.

Yet as I look back on her death, I do so with the certainty that at her time of greatest need, we all did the right thing. She was home, she had us, she had hospice care, and she had pain control. Work and our other obligations could wait, this was the time for us to gather and care for her. It was a passage of profound grief and profound learning. But at the same time, her death showed me how hard it can be to die and I hoped to never see someone I cared about suffer like that again. And I learned also that caring for the dying is all consuming. The hospice nurses taught us how to care for her but the long hours of caretaking fell on us as a family. And when I was diagnosed, those images played in my mind as I lay sleepless and ruminating in bed.

My father was selfless in taking care of my mother for the five years it took for the cancer to kill her. He lived for 13 years after my mother died. After she died he sold the house he had built and moved to a retirement community, he made new friends, he traveled and he continued his investing and reading.

He was eighty-six when he had a massive stroke. I believe he knew it was coming. He had perhaps had some minor strokes leading up to it that were mentioned but not discussed. What he did discuss was his friends who had had strokes and especially his friends' families who insisted that everything be done to keep them alive even if this was only possible in a hospital with multiple machines humming away to put fluid in for those who could not swallow, take fluid out for those who could no longer urinate, guess at the discomfort and unplanned wishes of those who could no longer speak, and ultimately die alone perhaps with only a kind nurse to sit with them in the last hours of their lives while their families carried on their lives often miles away. Or to be fair, the families and spouses that spent days, and weeks and months of their older years sitting by the bedside of a spouse or mother, or father who had worked hard, held a family together, shown character and compassion and love throughout their lives and now at the end of life were confined in a body that was no longer worthy of their lives.

My father's wishes, his demands, were clear: "Don't let that happen to me," he said.

And my brother and I had heard the plans every time we visited and even the threats of his anger and possibly revenge if we messed them up.

"If you do that to me, I will never forgive you."

"It's stupid, its unkind."

"And don't buy me a casket either. Cremate me. Scatter me among trees – I love trees. I have already made the arrangements. Here is the address for the funeral home. I wrote out the plans. There is a copy in this file here in this drawer. It is all organized."

I fantasized about him never forgiving me after he died. He was at most agnostic about an afterlife and he flatly said, "I can't do anything about it. When I'm dead I'll find out. I just need to live a good life." So, it seemed odd to think that he would have the ability to forgive or not forgive at that point. But it did put an image of a ghostly father in my mind, shaking his big fingers at me saying, "I told you not to do that, no machines."

When we went to his house after his stroke, while he was still in the hospital, we found that he had put his advanced care directive on the entry table. It could not be missed.

We took him home to die. His four grandchildren came to spend time with him. Even while he could not speak or move or swallow and was mostly sleeping, he seemed to recognize them.

He knew what he wanted and did not want. My father had a plan. It consisted of a large bottle of white tablets kept in the medicine cabinet of his bathroom in a house in the retirement community that never felt like his home.

When the hospice visiting nurse went through his medications with us, she looked at these pills and the question was written on her face. She did not even need to say it aloud.

"He had a plan," I said.

He died at home with hospice care and with my brother Barry and his wife Chris and Jim and me sitting vigil and all surrounding his bed with our hands on him at his last breath. He died as he asked to die, as he had written and told us. His death belonged to him. It was our role to protect him from excess measures, from unwanted visitors, from discomfort, from isolation. It was our role to be sure he had what he asked for. Yet at the end the choking sob again exploded from my core and at the same time I felt relief that it was over.

My mother-in-law, Mildred, died in her own home, with Jim and his sister at her side, in comfort, with care that only the wealthy can afford. After a broken hip and slowly accumulating dementia, her years of running a lumber business on her own after her beloved husband died young and her stewardship of every penny of her profits, allowed her to afford three years of care at home. She peacefully slipped away at the age of 92, one year before I was diagnosed. There were no hard decisions to make, no bankruptcy, no pain or suffering. There was only a life well lived in health until the end.

Even as we learn our values in life from our parents, we learn our values in death as well. Thinking about dying and thinking about death are two different things. My fears of dying cannot be understood without understanding the deaths I have been present for and participated in, my mother, my father and my mother-in-law. Each of them taught me something.

I was raised that you go to the hospital when you have something that can possibly be fixed — but that does not include dying. Death comes even when everyone, the professionals, the family and the patient are trying to save a life. The problem is telling the difference. People get trapped in the hospital with more and more machines, initially with the hope they will be well again. And then they are stuck, in a place they don't want to be, surrounded by people they don't know busily carrying out their tasks of blood samples and machine monitoring, and though their faces are smiling and concerned, they are not familiar. Even the best hospital professionals and staff are not family, they don't have that history or remembrance of that person at another time and another age. Too late, the family realizes the patient will not recover and will never go home. They cannot disconnect from the machines sustaining them, yet the end comes nevertheless.

I have seen this death also, the many life-sustaining machines despite the inevitability of death. Yet there is a place for this because sometimes it takes that level of medical care and those expert professionals to lessen the pain and discomfort of dying.

It is important to realize that a person can have a bad death at home or in the hospital. The fact of being at home, does not mean that there will be a good death. Home death puts a burden on the family and that is a burden not all families are able or willing to take on. When a person has a serious illness and death comes slowly, there are hard decisions of how to provide care over a long number of weeks and months. It is not simply a matter of saying, "I want to die at home in my own bed." Even with home hospice care, the burden and work is on whoever is providing care at home on an hourly and daily basis and that unrelenting need can be too much especially for elderly friends and family as well as for younger family with multiple responsibilities. Hospice visits provide professional monitoring and teaching about how to care for the bed-bound person. They help to acquire the equipment and medications needed to do that. But it is up to the caregivers to be consistent and present.

Caring for the terminally ill during the last months and weeks is wrenching and all consuming and in many cases the home cannot provide the resources that the dying person needs. With cancer, death is not sudden, preparations can be made, but the time period is uncertain, the expenses are unknown, the interference with work and with other family responsibilities especially if there are other sick family members and if children also need care, it all can make home care impossible. The end can be peaceful or painful. Each of these facts can add to the confusion of what is the best plan. Sometimes there is no plan and the path is just fallen into without direct intent. Only advance planning and discussions can ease this transition but those discussions are hard to enter for everyone. And in the worst case, even if there seems to be a plan, it can fall through, the caregiver can get sick as well. The bills might not be paid and the eligibility period may be exceeded so that with little notice, a new plan needs to be devised at the last minute.

We were fortunate. The plan was clear for my parents and for my mother-in-law, the wishes were discussed, the resources were available and we were able to provide the home care needed.

When I was diagnosed, there was no getting around the possibility that I could die from ovarian cancer. And, it is trite to say, "everyone dies." There is a lack of wisdom and deep thought in these two words.

As I have worked with patients with cancer, at times even while treatment is ongoing, when there has been a recurrence and a new treatment is tried, I have heard women say, "I just want this to be over." And there is an ambiguity in wanting to live but rejecting the conditions they must live with. Rejecting the uncertainty, the burden placed on others, the knowledge that nothing may work and that these end days are just a waiting game until they reject trying anything more.

It is the most profound transition and carries deep grief and confusion because it is often accompanied by deep relief for the failing body and those who stand watch. A sense of loss and a sense of relief at a burden lifted and suffering ended are present at the same time and for the same event. This is a confusing and guilt filled set of conflicting emotions. Those who care for the dying person must reconcile those opposite feelings in a way that brings peace and not shame.

Those lessons, those images of final days, and those decisions we make as caregivers become the focus of remembrances and rumination. I learned about good and bad endings and how to make the bad endings as bearable as possible. Often in the darkness of the night when sleep evaded me, I wished for my parents to be back, and in some mysterious way, I sought their spirit to teach me and protect me. And in those dark nights, I also knew that however I approached this would be the lessons for my own children and I felt I needed to get it right for them and they would need to get it right for me.

If only we could send messages to the universe, to God, to physicians and family that we want to go peacefully at home surrounded by those who love us most. Dying is part of life and it is unavoidable and the hope is that it does not come too young and that it is not too hard. The uncontrollability of illness and aging may not allow us that wish. But wish we will.

Lives are the same in two ways, they start with a birth and end with a death. What happens in between is the definition and meaning and importance of life. What happens in between is the learning and caring and purpose of a life. What happens in between are the people and the linkages and the love and the anger, and the separation and the coming together and the saying good-bye. When death comes it is a life well lived that brings comfort.

Chapter 26: And then Jackson Got Cancer

Seven years later, after I finished treatment, when Jackson was an aged 14-year-old, we noticed a hard lump on his chest, different from the fatty lumps that he had for several years. After a needle biopsy the diagnosis was soft tissue sarcoma.

"We can operate," the vet said, "but he is an old dog, maybe not such a good idea. He has about 3 months."

But three months later the lump seemed about the same. "We are survivors," I told him and he continued on, eating and stiffly following us from place to place and sometimes getting himself stuck in corners confused or unable to turn around. As we gently eased him out of the corner and settled him on his bed, he sunk down with an appreciative groan as though that was what he had been looking for. I wished I could have asked him what his wishes were. Would he have wanted surgery at that point or just the gentle care that we gave him?

A few months later there was an oozing sore on his belly. Again, we took him to the vet and learned he had a mast cell tumor.

"Let's schedule him for surgery," a different vet said, and we said "yes". But when we got home, we reconsidered and canceled.

"We will keep him as long as he continues eating," we decided. "We will know when it is time. But not yet."

But this tumor was aggressive and seemed to grow like a mushroom every day until we had to face the inevitable.

I stayed with him as the medications were given and quietly his heart stopped and my quiet comforting turned into a torrent of tears.

Months later, I still walked in the house and expected to be greeted. I expected to have Jackson next to me as I worked at my desk. When the bears came from the foothills to eat the avocados in our yard, Jackson would not be there to bark and warn me. The grandsons would now just be a twosome and not a threesome. The leftovers would go in the containers in the refrigerator until they were inedible and then go in the trash. I wouldn't be able to share cheese or ice cream with him.

I was blessed to have Jackson when I went through cancer. But, in the end, I needed to let him go. Chemo and surgery on an old dog don't make sense to me. But we do a kindness to dogs that we don't do for people. When dogs are dying, in pain, uncomfortable, and can't eat — we make decisions and we end their lives. We don't do that for people. We wouldn't do that for my mother even though we knew it was the end and she said she wanted to die. The heartbreak of seeking death for a dog was real and he left a vacant space, but somehow the decision felt right. But the heartbreak of seeing a person I loved die a miserable death will never leave me. I know the effort it took to care for my mother during her prolonged struggle fluctuating between dying and living. The consuming role for my father, the caregiver over several years, left no time for himself. Love of a person at the end of life, demands constant care not knowing when or how the end will come. But love of a dog demands just the opposite. I wondered which was kinder.

Cancer can be a trap with no way out but biding the time to see what happens. Will prayers be answered, will a reprieve be given, or will the worst images of death play out? And if those worst images become reality, what are the choices and who gets to make them? Who is the moral decision maker? Can rules be loosened without crossing the line and making death a matter of convenience for the living? And of course, it came full circle and the questions became all about myself and the decisions I might need to make if cancer came back.

Chapter 27: Expectations and Explanations

There are few diseases that elicit awkward comments to the extent that cancer does. It brings out the terror that people often try to hide but inevitably their words and actions belie their deeply rooted fear. Few people are ready to talk about cancer and stumble around looking for words. And worse, some disappear and avoid any contact.

People push expectations on those with cancer that are based on their own beliefs, needs and experiences, however misguided and distinct from the person with cancer. They are like the proselytizer at the door trying to convert me, the political pamphleteer trying to persuade me, or the car salesman trying to sell me, all of whom bring their own needs and wants to the interaction to achieve their own ends, and to leave knowing they have succeeded in their mission. And they want the interaction to be limited as though a box needed to be checked off and the conversation, however short and misguided, is sufficient to check that box, another soul saved, another car sold, another vote secured, another conversation ended.

Some comments veer towards the calamitous, toward words of pessimism and doom, and some veer toward the ridiculous.
" I hope you don't have too much pain."
"Everyone I knew with this disease died."
"I know you are sick but can you just finish this project?"

Alternatively, it brings out words of unrealistic optimism that everything will be alright. There are subterfuges that shadow discussions of cancer and ways in which cancer has been shrouded, sometimes in secrecy and sometimes in pretenses spun around it like pink cotton candy that has no substance, is artificially sweet and begins to disintegrate as soon as it is spun. Some talk in the abstract or in religious platitudes, the belief that there is a reason for everything or the belief that we are not given more than we can bear. For some it is the belief that God will save them and for others that, in death, God will meet them.

"Everything will be fine, you are strong."
"When I die, I hope I come back as a horse."
" It's Gods will and heaven is waiting"

It brings out the war analogy; that a fighting spirit, strength and toughness will lead to victory over cancer. Some people make boastful challenges, "This cancer tangled with the wrong person." "I am going to kick cancer's ass." But cancer is not a war. It is not an external enemy. What does that mean to kick cancer's ass? And what does it mean for those who do not survive? That as a warrior you failed? You weren't tough enough? You didn't try hard enough?

I found myself trying on the expectations that other people were convinced was the way to face cancer. Sometimes I found myself mouthing words I did not completely believe. I did not like the fighter metaphor and yet I accepted that others saw me fighting. Did I let their perceptions dominate the conversation in order to keep relationships and bonds that were more important to me than clarifying how I felt? Was I avoiding thinking and articulating the confusion, uncertainty, and also the resolve and determination that I really felt? Or was it simply that the process of being a cancer patient demanded so much physical and emotional reckoning that the ability to really feel and honestly say, "this is who I am, this is what I feel, these are my fears, these are my strengths and weaknesses, this is what I need from you now;" — that ability to self-perceive and articulate failed under that stress? I did not have the energy or desire or clarity to explain myself.

It does require grit to tolerate treatment but it also requires calmness, a slowing to allow time to heal, perhaps a meditation or a prayer to calm the mind, and a caring community of family and friends.

For me, the best way to get through this was to be determined but meditative, quiet, maybe reflective, and resilient. I adhered to the words I came to at the beginning: gratitude, integrity, and determination. On the worst days, those words continued to sustain me and bring me to the place of living despite my disease. I had little bravado except that I would tough out the treatment and learn to live the fullest life I could despite the uncertainty. So maybe that is a quiet bravado. Some days I felt certain I would survive. Some days the discouraging prognosis and the uncontrollability and fear of cancer overwhelmed me. And after treatment, at times I felt I was just waiting for the recurrence and steeling myself against that disappointment.

Joan Didion wrote the book, *The Year of Magical Thinking* about her remembrances of the death of her husband after a long marriage in which they together and separately wrote books and scripts. Together they fully experienced their life together through work, travel, and parenthood. Over cocktails and dinner in their own apartment, he died suddenly and quietly while she cooked dinner. And maybe because life could never be the same or because she wished it could be, she entered her period of magical thinking.

What is magical thinking? For my rational mind, magical thinking did not seem like a place I would go, and yet the magical thinking began. Lying in the bathtub with Epson salts and hot water and no hair, I would think about signs and deals. "If my CA-125 dropped by 50% at the next visit it would mean that I would be cured;" "If the bird flies off the wire I will be cured;" "if 100 people pray for me, I will be cured." Perhaps magical thinking in the face of a deadly disease is part of being human and part of maintaining hope. Perhaps it is part of being unable to confront mortality and to imagine oneself dead. Perhaps the religious spirit, the fighting spirit, and the unrealistic optimism are ways that magical thinking is at the core of being human and a way of avoiding a true discussion and engagement with the disease and the fear of the possibility of death that creeps closer day by day like a storm that you can see coming but cannot run fast enough to escape. Magical thinking may be helpful to slow the acceptance, to lessen the shock, to let the affected slowly adapt, adjust, and live on.

People with cancer go through a lonely experience. No one else could feel the physical assault or the petrifying fear that death may be near. The world would go on for the people I love, a beloved spouse may find love again, children would continue on with their lives and careers, grandchildren would forget, people would laugh and love and see the sunlight every day; but I would be gone. How could I process that?

For me the world stopped and the focus was limited and finite. It was a daily struggle for life to indeed go on. And it was a daily struggle to communicate because few people really wanted to talk about cancer and yet it interfered with all other discussions as well. I wanted to say "wait, something terrible is happening. You all need to pay attention. Stop what you are doing and focus on the trouble I am in." But that does not happen, it should not happen and at my best, I did not want it to happen. And though my illness filled my mind, there was also the desire to just be normal, to plan for holidays and travel and to not talk or think about cancer.

Sometimes people ask me questions about surviving cancer that make me feel like I should have learned important life lessons and I should be changed by it. People ask earnestly "How has cancer changed you?" I fear they are expecting me to have some wisdom about the state of the world, and me in it, that can be shared and give them an "Ah ha" moment. They have notions of a spiritual awakening, or a transformation of values.

Some are looking for stories of redemption like the Michael Milkin story. After being convicted of securities violations, and serving time in prison, he was diagnosed with cancer. When he was released he became a major donor to cancer research and endowed the George Washington University School of Public Health. Or maybe it is even the John McCain story. After a cancer diagnosis he saved the Affordable Care Act to provide health insurance to millions despite previously opposing it.

Some people want to see anger.

"You must be really pissed off."
"You worked to prevent cancer and now you have it, so unfair."
"This is so unfair."

But that was not how I felt. Why did this happen to me? It happened. Nobody knows why. Fair or unfair is immaterial. Or perhaps they expected me to be so depressed by the whole prospect of having cancer that I would not be able to experience joy again. Amazingly, some people seem to want to hear that. But I never felt that way either.

How has cancer changed me? Cancer left me with a profound awareness of my mortality. Yet I could not live happily if that was the recurring and constant awareness of my life. I wanted to still plan for the future. But I also knew it could all end in the not-too-distant future. Bringing the conflicting awareness of the end and the future into balance, is like swimming in a rip tide. At some level you let the dangerous tide carry you because it is too strong to swim against. If you struggle to swim against it you will become exhausted and drown. It takes you out further until the distance seems impossible. And then it lets you go and you must slowly swim to shore on a diagonal line to arrive at a different place than you started or aimed for, far from the umbrella and towels that you carelessly left on the distant beach. And when you get back to that place where you left your towels, you lie exhausted, grateful to be alive and soon you begin to plan for the drive home and dinner.

That awareness of mortality can suppress joy and planning and useful work. I struggled against this. But through all of that, there is also the reality of life that cannot be eroded or destroyed by such fear.

Humans plan. That is in our nature. With cancer, we check our plans. I had a tooth that needed a crown. But what was the point of getting a crown if I was not going to survive longer than the tooth or the crown?

I had an old car that was giving me trouble and I no longer trusted it. But what was the point of buying another car? And if I did buy one should it be cheap and old and just enough to get me through two years?

Did cancer change how I saw the world, how I live my values, how I experience my own tribulations in relationship to the tribulations of others? Do I appreciate life more than I did before? These may be the expected changes, the stereotype, and for me that particular stereotype fit. There is a part of me that sees suffering more clearly and invests in kindness more fully. There is a part of me that cares more deeply and speaks more directly. The changes are subtle but I do feel them.

There is a notion that only by being so tried can a person truly appreciate life and learn to live life to the fullest. You see this all of the time in cancer testimonials – those who feel they are a better person after cancer. It sweetens the devastation of cancer. I don't think I see the flowers as more beautiful and when I stop to smell the roses, they smell about the same. Still, I am very aware of how fortunate I am to be here to smell them. I remember to be grateful that I can take a long walk, that I can kayak, and so much more. I live my life with more gratitude and that gratitude propels me to want to help others perhaps more than I might have otherwise. It counteracts selfishness and self-absorption. At some level it also makes me see foolishness, selfishness and dishonesty in others and in myself, such that I can't excuse it. It is a strange mix of greater patience with those who have great needs and few resources, and greater impatience with those who have much and give little.

I have heard people say that cancer made them a better person. I think cancer can bring out and accentuate the values that were already there whether that is generosity or selfishness, optimism or pessimism, strength or weakness, foolishness or wisdom, kindness or cruelty. Cancer cannot radically change a personality but it does reveal who you are. People bring to cancer whatever they have brought to life and if they are fortunate, they grow in compassion, understanding and patience for others who are facing a daunting challenge. It did not change who I am but it did transform considerations and reactions and change my perceptions of myself and what is possible. It changed my ability and desire to reach out to others facing such challenges with patience and without judgment. I believe I have grown with this experience, as does anyone who faces death and somehow survives through science and the grace of God.

I am able to carry out a healthy life, hiking, kayaking, playing Scrabble with my grandkids, watching them learn to surf, cheering at their sports events, and teaching them how to bake cookies and how to play poker. But despite the growth I have experienced, if anyone were to ask me if I am thankful for having gone through this – the answer is a certain and unequivocal "NO." I am thankful for surviving.

PART V: MILESTONES OF RECOVERY

Chapter 28: Get Out, Get Moving

When I hike there are milestones that tell me how far I have walked. They tell me whether I have gone longer or shorter distances than before and whether I have met my goals. And each of the hikes I regularly do in the San Gabriel Mountains has a different milestone. There is the first stream crossing, the first look-out point, the power lines, the place where the trail divides, the place where the trail gets steep or levels out, and if it is a loop trail, the place where I end up back where I started.

"Recovery" is such a simple word for a long process. It is used to describe those with illnesses and those with addictions. For addicts or alcoholics, it is prefaced by the word "in," as in "in recovery," and this seems to acknowledge the uncertainty of consistent progress.

In contrast, people with illnesses are seen as recovering or recovered, "I was sick and now I am well." Either that or the unwanted words "never recovered."

But I stutter-stepped my way to recovery. I was "in recovery" for a long time. It is a path, a process, a passage of time. It implies twists and turns, maybe set-backs and unexpected strengths and weaknesses, possible disappointments, losses and gains. It is not a gate one simply walks through from illness to health. It is more like a hike and it takes effort and perseverance and a fair amount of luck.

Recovery meant getting back to where I started, with increased wisdom perhaps. I wanted to get back to what I valued before cancer. More and new experiences might follow, but simply reclaiming and taking up where I left off, that was the first challenge.

I started babysitting my grandsons again.
I resumed riding my horse beyond just walking.
I went back to work.

I walked and I waited.

About two months after chemo ended I could see that I was getting some slight fuzzy hair growing back. What a relief. After eight months of hiding in hats, now I really couldn't wait to get out of them. "Look. Hair," I said, pointing to about 1/8 inch of new growth. "Hair!"

By October 2011, I was close to finishing my bevacizumab infusions. I ached mentally and emotionally to leave the protection of my home and the confinement of illness. I ached to make everything normal, to remember and regain my body.

I had not driven further than 25 miles from home since I got sick. I knew I needed to break through the chains of worry and regain my independence, to get in the car and drive somewhere alone beyond my familiar routes.

When my friend Nicki said she was going RVing with her husband George to Morro Bay, and my friend Bonnie who lived near the bay invited me to stay with her, it was the perfect opportunity to explore the bay and connect with old friends. I had worked with Nicki and Bonnie on various research projects involving cancer and AIDS. Both of them had moved out of the LA area and I had not seen either of them since I was diagnosed.

Bonnie worked as a Physician's Assistant in the AIDS clinic early in the epidemic before there was a treatment. Years before we had explored the wildflowers on the Carrizo Plain. I waited while she carefully set up her camera tripod and her reflective screens. She waited for the breeze to die down and then she took perfect pictures of the California poppies. Taking quick photos, I had hiked off only to come back to wait some more and to admire how a serious photographer worked.

When we first met in 1980, Nicki was a single parent with kids in junior high school and high school while my kids were in elementary school. One of her daughters broke the gender barrier and was the first girl to play in the boys Little League in Pasadena. Nicki's son had been diagnosed with a brain tumor in elementary school and he died in his late twenties. She grieved for the loss of his life and the loss of what his life could have been. And as an oncology nurse, she also understood what I was going through. She was a source of advice and a touchstone for me.

A drive to Morro Bay was a reasonable 4-hour challenge. I hoped to kayak on the bay. The last time I had kayaked was on Yellowstone Lake just before I was diagnosed. I was worried about my fitness but also confident because rental kayaks are broad and stable to keep beginners from falling out. I tried to convince Bonnie that her photography would be amazing from a kayak perspective but she had seen a video of a seal hauling itself on the front of a kayak and decided that she would have none of it.

The Morro Bay State Park nestles against the bay. When the campgrounds along the coast cleared out from the summer tourists, Nicki and George arrived with their RV and their canoe strapped on top.

It was windy and the water was choppy as we started out and I wondered if I was being too ambitious, following them as they canoed out in front of me. "Keep going " I told myself, "This is important, keep up … fight back, reclaim your life. " I was concentrating hard and despite the chill in the air, I was sweating as I kayaked. We headed south into the wetlands that lead off the bay, the water became less choppy, and my confidence returned. Now instead of just trying to keep up, I began to focus on my surroundings and to see the magnificence of the bay.

Morro Bay is on the Pacific flyway, a stopover for migratory birds. I had consulted my *Sibley Field Guide to Birds of Western North America* before starting out with the notion that I would be able to identify birds on the bay. Morro Bay has a bird festival in January and over 200 species have been identified. There was little hope that I could distinguish many of them. Still there were some that were familiar. The Black Oystercatchers were wading in the water with their distinctive black feathers, long orange beaks, and bright orange eyes that remind me of Halloween. Sitting in my kayak, the Great Blue Herron was taller than me and looked directly down its spike-like beak at me as though judging my vulnerability. I felt an unnerving shudder and found myself paddling faster. The Great White Egrets and the smaller Snowy Egrets dotted the marshy wetlands often flying up and treating us to their graceful swoop and landing. I struggled to remember as I went past wading birds, whether the Avocets or the Curlews had the upturned or the downturned beaks or whether the Godwits or the Whimbrels had the straight beaks.

Large California sea lions were grouped on the banks of the meandering tidal inlets. They could easily have knocked us out of our little boats, but they just seemed content to bark at us as we went by. They seemed to be the Labrador Retrievers of the bay, good natured, yet asserting that I was a stranger trespassing on their property. The younger ones swam out, popped their heads up and took a long look at me with their dark eyes and then followed my kayak reminding me of Bonnie's worry about them climbing aboard.

As the afternoon went on, the tide began to go out and the bay became shallower as we headed back. My paddle was hitting sand as the kayak was gliding just inches above the bottom. The inlets I had been in were now unpassable and I headed toward the center of the channel looking through incoming fog for the tiny dock where I had started. Though some smaller structures seemed to melt into the misty air, the Morro Rock stood out as my navigation point.

I knew I would not get lost despite the fog, but I felt cocooned in my little kayak. The silence of the afternoon wrapped around me and was at once exciting and also frightening. Solitude in nature is both strengthening and intimidating. The smallness of my body against the magnitude of the water and the thickness of the air challenged my now tired muscles to paddle back to the dock. When I pulled alongside the dock my legs were cold and seemed locked in place, unable to bend and my arms were aching. I could not get out of the kayak without dumping myself in the water. Graciously, the young man at the rental booth helped heave me up to sitting on the edge of the dock and eventually I was able to unwind my legs and hobble away until my legs and feet returned to normal.

I was regaining my footing. I was taking back my life from cancer. I was pushing back on fear. I was allowing the healing of nature to work its magic on my assaulted body and troubled thoughts. I was engaging in joy.

By January 2012 I had just finished my bevacizumab infusions. It was time to celebrate the end of treatment even though I could not ignore the threat of recurrence, I also knew that I needed to do something to put a period at the end of that chemo sentence and experience something that would break me out of the focus on treatment.

It may not seem an obvious choice, but I was drawn to the bellow of the elephant seals. I had seen them once before along the central coast of California. They come ashore from San Simion up to Año Nuevo just above Santa Cruz. They are most numerous around Valentine's Day when elephant seals are looking for their sweethearts and mostly looking for sex. The elephant seals return from their migration to battle and to breed. It seemed like the perfect road trip. My children, children-in-law, grandchildren, Jim and I all met in Santa Cruz with plans to see the seals and the Monterey Bay aquarium and then to head south stopping at tide pools on the way back home.

Año Nuevo is a point that sticks out into the Pacific Ocean and is now a California State Park especially designated to protect the elephant seals during their breeding. Guides lead groups to see them, and to keep everyone far enough away so as not to disturb the seals natural inclinations.

The males are enormous with a formidable proboscis and powerful teeth. When they are ready to breed they have battles, rearing up to as full a height as they can manage with their considerable weight and then smashing into each other to establish dominance. They get gashed and bloodied until one of them yields and galumphs off to find a lesser foe to take on.

The bachelors are half grown males that hang around in the water just off shore poking their wandering eyes and big noses comically up from the water like a pack of leering adolescents. They scan the beaches to see if perhaps a large bull male is asleep, allowing them to sneak ashore and mate with one of his females while he snoozes. But when the bull male awakens and finds the egregious sexual assault by a younger intruder, he quickly chases the young bachelor away. But the younger Casanova never stops scanning other harems for available females on his escape.

The females seem to ignore it all. Many have pups beside them looking like small dark blimps. The pups try hard to get out of the way of the big males who seem eager to breed with the moms shortly after recovery from birthing. The pups need to be alert to avoid getting crushed by the males who seem impervious to their presence.

The walk was a few miles out to the tip of Año Nuevo and back along the trails. The day was cold and perfect. Though there may have been other ways to celebrate finishing treatment, this trip with the wind, water, family, a hike, and the chance to witness the life cycle of the seals was my best wish.

Life cycle seemed to be the theme of this trip. The mating, the birthing and the nursing, the battling for dominance, and the young seals challenging the old. It was all right in front of me. The seals made it so apparent that this is the natural and inevitable story of life. The animal world shows often contradictory ways in which old age plays out, the wolf packs that wait for the elderly and the reindeer herds that move on allowing the elderly to be left behind and the first to go. But it was also in front of me with my grandchildren, now five of them, from six months to four years old. I was in that matriarchal space. The matriarch has much to give and to teach but at some point, that would end and that role would go to the next generation. It has always been such.

I have a picture from that day that I use in my public talks. It shows all of us with the Año Nuevo point and the Pacific Ocean behind us. On the beach are huge grey lumps, the elephant seals, exhausted from their travels and their mating. I was exhausted at the end of the three mile walk but also, I felt victorious. That soon after treatment ended, the unknown was still ahead and I was thinking about the lifecycle. I was looking forward and pushing against uncertainty.

Chapter 29: Bugs in my Ear

A while after finishing treatment, I began to notice a ringing in my left ear and the entire left side of my brain. Two sounds really, a low rumbling thrumming that sometimes seemed like a pulsing of my heart and a higher pitched ringing static. When I first experienced these sounds it was mild. Over time it increased to the point that I was imprisoned by it. In the middle of the night, I would awake and the sound was so loud that I wondered if the house smoke alarms were going off only to realize that the noise was from inside my head.

There were days when this ringing, called tinnitus, sounded like the small bells used by a Hari Krishna band of chanting shaved-head, saffron-clothed men asking for money on the street corner. There were days it sounded like high pitched static or insects like cicadas or a beehive lodged inside my head. And there were days that I could not tell the difference between the crickets outside and the insect sounds inside my head, and I would need to ask Jim if he was hearing crickets also. It was exhausting and I wanted to beg for it to stop every minute of the day. But it didn't. I tried every remedy I could think of. The hot baths that soothed the chemo side effects did not ease the tinnitus. I tried refraining from certain foods and drinks to see if that would help. I tried going for massage. I tried various over-the-counter medications hoping they might help. And while relaxation exercises had worked so well going through cancer treatment, it did nothing for the tinnitus. It was difficult to be in crowds. The sounds in my head dominated casual conversation. Walking helped a bit, sitting seemed worse, and lying down was worst of all. I began to dread going to bed at night. Sleep, for many months, was nearly impossible.

After cancer, every unusual twinge got linked back to my cancer, whether I got a stomachache or a headache or felt fatigued. The question was always there, "Is it back?" I told one friend that I was living with optimism on one shoulder and fear on the other. The ringing made me fear that I had metastases to my brain.

Agustin said he was certain it was not brain metastases, but after several weeks he agreed to order a CT of my neck and head. Thankfully, he was right.

Tinnitus can occur after taking chemotherapeutic drugs particularly the platinum-based drugs like the carboplatin. These drugs are called ototoxic which just means they are toxic to the auditory nerve and other parts of the ear. I have talked with other women who have been on chemotherapy and several have had either some loss of hearing or tinnitus to varying degrees. It is a common complaint, and it is often passed off as unimportant and a problem to be tolerated.

I went to an otolaryngologist to see if he could help me with this. The hearing test showed no loss of hearing.

"You have tinnitus," he said.

"I know" I said suppressing the cynical words "tell me something I don't know."

"I think you may be depressed," he said.

"No, I don't think that is it," I said wondering how he reached that diagnosis without asking me any of the questions usually asked on a depression screening interview. Questions I had asked many times in my research. Was he suggesting the tinnitus was caused by depression? If people with tinnitus were also depressed, it seemed more likely to me that the unrelenting buzzing and static of tinnitus caused the depression rather than the other way around. Nor did he ask about the chemo that I had received that might have caused this. I volunteered this information but he seemed unimpressed.

"What can you do for me?" I asked.

"You will need to learn to live with it," he said, "it is common in older people." He stood up ready to leave and finish his five-minute visit.

Tinnitus for him: common, boring, no cure.

Tinnitus for me: torturous, unrelenting, interfering with my activities.

To ease the sound, I walked back and forth in my house. Jackson followed me and I would hear the click click of his nails on the wood floor to the point that I would yell at him to go lie down. The clicking and the sound of buzzing bees and high pitch static filled my head with unrelenting noise. My frustration was let loose on Jackson who held no grudges.

I consulted a neurologist who gave me a full battery of neuropsychological tests that I recognized from my own prior research. I was told to walk on a line, touch my nose with my eyes closed, stand on one foot, remember words, alternate numbers and letters, and perform memory tests to determine my neurologic function. I had used the very same tests in my studies of neuropsychological effects in women with HIV/AIDS.

"What is the capital of Delaware?" he asked at the end.

"Dover" I said. The test was over.

"How did you know Dover was the capital of Delaware?" Jim asked later.

"Lucky," I said, "he just picked one that I remembered."

The neurologist suggested an MRI but it did not show the cause of tinnitus – no pinched nerves that he could see and no tumors pushing on nerves either. He prescribed muscle relaxants that did not help the tinnitus but dulled my thinking and made me drowsy. This was not the solution I was hoping for and I stopped taking them and continued to tolerate the noise in my head.

As the months went by, if I had a day that seemed even slightly better I would tell myself that it was getting better and I just needed to wait it out. If I had a day that was worse, I would wonder how I was going to live with this. What if this was going to continue for the remainder of my life?

Tinnitus is common among the aged but it is also the leading disability of young people discharged from the military. I thought about all of the young service men and women who were coming home from war zones and having tinnitus on top of the PTSD and I wondered if anyone was studying this as a contributing factor to the high suicide rates. I began to understand how an unrelenting injury, or pain, or tinnitus or PTSD could contribute to suicide among these young vets.

The tinnitus has lessened considerably over the years. The noise volume has lessened from the persistent sense of a beehive in my head to a tolerable constant and still annoying static. Now I can divert my attention away from it and function normally but it never stops.

I can't be sure that the tinnitus was caused by the chemo, but it is likely that it was. Tinnitus was the only side effect of chemo that drove me to tears and despite every solution I tried, I was unable to control it. Was it neuropathy of the auditory nerve similar to the neuropathy and tingling in my feet? Was it the loss of cilia in my inner ear similar to hair loss? Even these simple questions don't seem to have answers. The impact on me was not heard by others and the complaining as they say, "fell on deaf ears."

Chapter 30: Time for a Change

My career was an important part of my life and I enjoyed and valued it immensely. I achieved a leadership position in the School of Medicine as a full professor. I taught graduate students for over thirty years and served on many dissertation committees. I taught undergraduates for twenty years. I competed for and been awarded research grants from the National Institutes of Health, the American Cancer Society and the Centers for Disease Control. I received awards for my research and I received a teaching award for mentoring junior faculty. USC awarded me the faculty Lifetime Achievement Award and UCLA School of Public Health selected me for the Alumni Hall of Fame Award. I had a fulfilling and challenging career.

But it was clear to me that I did not want to continue to apply for research grants or to run large multiyear studies like those I had run in the past. Nor did I want to move up the chain of administrative leadership. Gradually I shed my responsibilities, transferred my responsibilities to others and retired in 2014 four years after my diagnosis and a few months after I turned sixty-five years old and qualified for Medicare.

Retirement is like other transitions in life. It was a challenge to shed that identity of professor that I had worked so hard and so long to obtain. I had trepidations, even though I knew that I did not want to continue doing most of what my work entailed. Retirement is like college graduation when everyone asks, "What are you going to do now?" I have images of Dustin Hoffman being asked this in *The Graduate* and he seemed clueless. I did not feel clueless. I had plans, some small and some large. But the unknown was my health. My work and my colleagues had helped me get through cancer. What if I had a recurrence and no work? It would feel isolating. But still, clinging to work for that reason would have been clinging to fear and that I did not want to do either.

I wanted to start piano lessons and learn Beethoven sonatas.
I had piles of books to read and a library card.

I had friends I rarely visited and many who were retiring.
I had topographical maps for hikes I wanted to take.
I had shelves and drawers full of art materials.
I had five grandchildren (and the year after I retired the sixth was born).
I had ambitions of addressing societal problems.
And I had tents for camping and skis that had been gathering dust.

It seemed there was no end to the possibilities. And as emeritus professor, I could keep my linkages with the University. Retirement felt like a new beginning and although I missed my colleagues and the identity my career invited, I found retirement opened up new doors and explorations.

Chapter 31: It's not About the Calendar

There are major milestones in recovery that are tied to the calendar of months and years since diagnosis. Data is reported often for survival rates at two years and five years. When I passed the two-year mark without a recurrence, I looked at the published survival curves and I realized that I needed to actually get to three years before the survival curve flattened out. And when I passed that I began to look to the five-year mark. Five years is the milestone for most survival data reports.

August 2020 marked my tenth year since diagnosis. But still, I continue to look over my shoulder to make sure the cancer is not following me.

Fear of recurrence is almost unavoidable after a diagnosis of cancer. Small changes or twinges in my abdomen cause me to go on alert. If my stomach looks distended more than normal, it makes me wary because that can be a symptom of ovarian cancer. I review my diet and see if there are other reasons, too much hummus or chili perhaps?

There are 15 million cancer survivors in the United States and I would bet that every one of them has experienced fear of recurrence. It is something I still hold even at ten years since I was diagnosed. The chances were very low that I would survive especially without a recurrence and further treatment, and I knew that from the start. The fear of recurrence and even the expectation that cancer could come back nags at the mind of every cancer patient even those with an excellent outlook at diagnosis. It is a fear that some dwell on and talk about and for others an awareness that is shunned and ignored. But always it is there and the more I can emerge from that shadow the more I can live a more purposeful life. Yet I don't know any ovarian cancer survivor who does not hold her breath before her follow-up visits, before she knows the CA-125 number or the scan results.

Agustin has moved to another university but my health care has been seamless. I am now followed by my friend and colleague Dr. Darcy Spicer who I have known even longer than Agustin. My visits are a combination of medical monitoring and sharing stories of the events of our lives.

Nevertheless, when I go for my annual follow-up visit, I feel the tension build and the sleepless night before is almost inevitable. I know women who say they become grumpy and solitary. If the CA-125 ticks up, even if it stays in the normal range, there is worry and fear. And when I get a normal lab result I put it out of my mind until the next visit only to go through the same process again. I wonder when I will ever say that I am done with ovarian cancer. It is this way for me after ten years. It is much worse for women who have had a recurrence.

Advanced ovarian cancer with no recurrence and few long-term effects is unusual. It turns out that I am an "exceptional responder." There is a perplexing reality about cancer. At every stage there are people who survive and people who don't. Even given the exact same treatment, there are differences in how the tumor responds. For the past 20 years, carboplatin and Taxol have been given to almost all women with ovarian cancer. Yet the outcomes are often very different. Why is that?

Within the last five years a new class of drugs called PARP Inhibitors (PARPi) have been developed. These drugs are based on an understanding of the genetic errors related to a biological process called Homologous Repair Deficiency that leads to ovarian cancer. What is important here is that these drugs make use of a deeper understanding of cancer to specifically target DNA mutations. These drugs have been subjected to clinical trials and are now being used in first-line and recurrent disease. While standard chemotherapy is a blunt force medication designed to kill cells, these new drugs are tailored. Initially PARPi were restricted to women with BRAC1/2 mutations but are now used for women without these mutations also. More drugs will come. Unfortunately, at this time, immune therapies that have been effective with other cancers (notably melanoma), have not been effective against ovarian cancer. However, as research continues and new strategies to use the immune system to kill cancer cells are developed, this may well change in the future.

Responding to treatment means there was a nexus between the treatment and the particularities of the cancer. Does the cancer succumb when those little baggies of chemo are infused or does it ignore the chemo and continue to grow? There are mutations in the cancer cells that determine whether the cancer cells will respond to chemotherapy. This response is determined by the biological characteristics of any particular cancer. Were the particular genetic mutations in my cancer cells unusually susceptible to chemo? Did the chemo allow the immune system to attack it? The biology of cancer is still being unlocked. Studies are ongoing to answer all of these questions.

The challenge of cancer research today – is to develop new therapies that will be specific for the mutations that are present in the cancer cells of any particular patient. This is what is meant by "individualized therapy."

I often think back on that time when I was in treatment and reflect on what gave me strength and what gave me not just hope but optimism. My physicians had seen other women survive ovarian cancer. They did not offer dire warnings that would have taken away my hope. I had confidence in them, and to that extent my mind was at ease. I was otherwise healthy and active before my diagnosis. During chemo I continued to walk the trails, at a slower pace for sure, but still walking was a daily objective – except for those days when the chemo kept me pinned to the sofa. Did the calm of knowing, trusting and being comfortable talking with my care team, and continuing to exercise contribute in some way to me being an exceptional responder?

Again, I wonder, "Why am I an exceptional responder?" It is not because I fought harder, it is not because I was otherwise healthier, it is not because I deserve to live more than others, it is not because I had greater faith. Was it the support of family and friends? Was it exercise? Was it feeling safe and comfortable with those who were managing my chemo and surgery? Was it some rare perfect fit between the chemo and the mutations in my ovarian tumor cells? I was lucky, the cancer cells in my tumors succumbed to the chemo I was given and the tumor died. Right now, the exact reasons are unknown but some day the answers will be clear. I believe those reasons are knowable. For women like me, with ovarian cancer, and for others with difficult cancers, the breakthroughs have been slow in coming, but they will come.

Chapter 32: Hiking and Camping

Hiking and camping became part of my recovery. A few years after I finished treatment Jim and I camped with our camping buddies Juliann and Maggie in Death Valley. It was our first camping trip since my diagnosis and also our first time camping in Death Valley. The weather was cool and it was a good time to go. We took short hikes to see the almost extinct pup-fish and the dunes as well as the salt plains in the center of the valley. We drove to Zabriskie Point and took pictures. Although the pictures made it look like we had climbed a peak, in fact the parking lot was not far away. On the way home we were caught in the traffic coming back to LA from Las Vegas and I was glad to prefer camping to casinos. It was our first camping trip since I was diagnosed.

The following summer we all went to Sequoia and Kings Canyon National Parks. Kings Canyon is similar to the Yosemite Valley but with fewer people and cars along the pristine river flowing through the steep rock wall canyon. The giant trees of Sequoia were logged over a century ago but since 1890 those groves are left untouched and protected. The oldest tree is estimated to be 3200 years old which was enough to make me feel like a speck in time, and just one in a long line of people responsible to protect them from further capricious damage.

Jim and I brought our Coleman canvas cabin tent that we bought when we were first married in 1969. It is a far cry from the pop-up tents now sold. It is made of heavy canvas, there are support poles and ridge poles to put together and to fit into grommets. It takes us about 20 minutes to put it up. Once up, it feels like a little cabin with enough head-room to stand and enough space for a queen-size blow-up mattress and two collapsible chairs. There were no other tents in the campground that looked like the same vintage, and Juliann said it looked like a MASH tent, if only it had a red cross on the side. This trip felt like a nostalgic milestone.

Now that we are both "mostly" retired, Alexandra and I hike in the San Gabriel Mountains once a week. We listen to the woodpeckers and see their holes drilled into a particular grove of trees along the way as we try to spot their red heads obsessively pecking into the trees. We have seen deer many times coming down canyon walls to the stream and up the other side. Bobcats have crossed our paths. We have seen the streams dry out in the summer and fill up in the winter, we have walked on rocks across streams and hiked to waterfalls and to look-out points. We have passed homeless people who use the National Forest as a home base, safer than the city streets, but their cooking fires a potential threat to wildfires in dry weather. We talk about politics and medicine, theater, and family and these conversations have been going on for nearly forty years.

*

The summer of 2018, I enrolled in a printmaking workshop at the Idyllwild Art Camp, in a beautiful mountain community a two-hour drive from my home. I had first noticed my vague symptoms at a printmaking class in Colorado in 2010 and this return to art camp felt like another milestone of recovery. For prior workshops I had rented a cabin with artist friends or rented a dorm room when I went alone. Another friend told me about a beautiful county campground a mile from the art studios and I decided to reserve a campsite. I bought the meal plan at the art camp, to avoid cooking and washing dishes for a week. "Camping and art, what could be better?" I thought.

I pitched my backpacking tent, which was orders-of-magnitude smaller than our cabin tent. The first night, Saturday, the campsite rangers led a family education program. They said they did not see bears in the area but there was a pack of coyotes in the area that were shy of humans and well fed due to sufficient numbers of rabbits and ground squirrels. "The coyotes won't bother people" the ranger assured us, which set my mind at ease, "but if you leave food out they will steal it."

The campground was filled on Saturday night with many large loud groups who respectfully settled down by 10 pm. Sunday night the campground was about half full, and by Monday night it was almost empty. At night after eating and hearing an artist talk or listening to a music performance at the art camp, I went back to my little tent and crawled inside with my lantern to read. The nights felt long as I read through two books in the five nights.

I had never camped by myself before. My uncertainty and caution on the first night gradually gave way to confidence and boredom by the last night. I have read *Wild* by Cheryl Strayed and admired and fantasized about her independence and courage, in camping and hiking the Pacific Crest Trail alone. While I will never do that, this did force a certain amount of solitude in nature but with amenities. It was a lovely morning experience to roll out of a sleeping bag and crawl out of a tent, greet the morning and the busy birds, and walk on a path through tall pine trees to the coin operated showers. Having filled my thermos with hot tea the evening before, the first hour of the day I spent reading or sketching at my campsite picnic table before heading over to the art camp cafeteria to enjoy breakfast and conversation with other artists.

At the end of the week, I rolled up my sleeping bag, deflated my mattress, pulled up my tent stakes, collapsed my tent, rolled it up and put it in a duffle, and packed my lantern, flashlight, and books back in the car before heading to the art studios for my last day of workshop. At the end of the day, after goodbyes and promises to stay in touch, I drove down the mountain enjoying the views out over Palm Springs.

I had found that there were still doors to open and walk through. It was a small challenge but it was beyond my normal and that was a confidence builder. Even if I never camp alone again, I know I can if I want to. It was part of my belief that walking is medicine and walks in nature would heal my body and my mind. Even if I never hike the Pacific Crest trail with a backpack like Cheryl Strayed, I have experienced the healing solitude of nature.

In 2018, Juliann got certified as a Sierra Club hike leader. The first hike she led was to Gray's Peak at Big Bear Lake, seven miles round trip and 1200-foot elevation gain. I thought I would not be able to accomplish this and would sign-out and return to the base early. But the "sweep", who is the person who hikes in the last place to be sure that nobody gets left behind, talked with me and told me stories of his hiking experiences all the way up the mountain. Because I was out of breath most of the way I could barely respond. Thankful for his tales, I completed the hike with only sore feet. This proved to me that the limitations I had put on myself, what I thought I could do, were less than what I could actually do.

The next day I turned seventy years old and I marked eight years since starting on cytotoxic chemotherapy.

Chapter 33: How Long has it been Since…?

When I tell people that I have had cancer, it is not unusual for them to ask "How long has it been since you were diagnosed?"

"August 2010," easy to remember.

Some ask, "How long has it been since you had surgery?"

"February 2011." Seared in my brain. The 17th to be exact.

But one day I was stumped. Instead of asking me to answer one of the dates that I won't forget and can't forget even if I wanted to, someone asked me something different. When I said I am writing about having a bad cancer, she asked, "How long has it been since you were cured?"

I felt like she asked me a trick question. I did not know how to answer. Was it a question where the attempt to be encouraging was imbedded in what pretended to be a genuine question? Was it how she perceived cancer – a disease you get then get over? Did she think I looked healthy enough to appear cured? Or did I lead her to ask it in that way because of how I speak about it?

"I had cancer" - (always past tense).

"When I was sick" – (past tense again).

I do at times think "I was sick, and now I am well."

But I was unsure how to answer. In truth, in the years since I was diagnosed, she was the first person to ask me that question in that way and it caused me to reflect on what that question meant to me and whether I believed it was true.

"How long has it been since I was cured?"

Was I cured after 18 weeks of carboplatin and Taxol when the CA-125 dropped to normal levels?

Was it after surgery, when the last identifiable micro-speck of cancerous cells was cut out?

Was it at 16 months after diagnosis when bevacizumab treatment finished and I went to see the elephant seals still worried that it might come back?

Was it at three years, when the survival curves begin to flatten out?

Was it at five years, when I went kayaking?

Or maybe at nine years when I went skiing?

We only know about "cure" with the passage of time.

Do I feel "cured" now? Am I afraid to say it because I fear I might jinx my recovery?

Sometimes I say quietly to myself, "I think I am done with this. I think it is behind me now, a lot of time has passed, I am beyond the elbow in the survival curve where the line flattens out like the bottom of a ski slope."

I have never said out loud to another person, "I am cured." I doubt that I ever will. Because there is that uncertainty; I have met women where it has come back years later. But I have also met women who have survived much longer than me.

When I finished treatment, I set a rule for myself. It was a logic rule that the left side of my brain conjured up and I tried to force into all the fear centers of my brain. It went like this: "If I spend these healthy days worrying about cancer coming back and it never does – then I have wasted my healthy life foolishly. If I spend these healthy days worrying about cancer coming back and it does come back some time in the future - then I have still wasted these healthy days foolishly." And I reflect again on what I want to do now that I have this time and this future that I was afraid I would not have.

I wonder if the answer can be that I just want to live, to love, to enjoy, and to do whatever gives my life meaning. I don't want to hold back.

Loving, enjoying, finding meaning – all of these offer a myriad of opportunities that bring to mind my six grandchildren, national parks, painting and piano, books and learning, friends and theatre. But also, because I am so grateful to have survived, I have become an advocate for ovarian cancer research and the women who have it. My answer involves all of these.

So, what did I answer when she asked me "How long has it been since you were cured?"

I said, "I don't know, but I choose to live like I am cured."

Chapter 34: Camp: A Community of Women

Camp Mak-A-Dream in Gold Creek Montana, is an hour outside of Missoula. All summer long camp is filled with children with cancer but in the spring and fall cancer camp is for adults, and one week is for women with ovarian cancer. It is here that women who don't know anyone else with this disease meet others who share it and feel part of a community of women. It is our turn to ride the zip line, hike the butte, climb the climbing wall, tell jokes, share, and cry and know we are surrounded with new friends who carry the same burden.

In the fall of 2017, I volunteered to give a talk on cancer research and to teach in the art room. I am a hybrid participant, a researcher with ovarian cancer who in retirement is a patient advocate and an artist. It seemed like the perfect fit.

I met two women on the plane into Missoula headed for the camp. Tall like me, they looked lean and healthy and had been there before. One from Texas and one from Reno, Nevada – they met a few years before and reunited at camp to continue their friendship and enjoy a week of fun. One, a former Spanish and German teacher was now a "peak bagger"; she and her husband were climbing the peaks of Nevada and beyond. I immediately saw that I wouldn't be the fittest person at camp and instead of needing to inspire others with my recovery and ability to move forward, I would be inspired by others.

The first night of camp began with an introductory circle and we gathered in the large community room. Sixty-five women with ovarian cancer, some in remission, some just finished chemo, some in treatment, some with recurrences and some without – those called the "one-and-done." Some wore hats, some wore scarves, some had buzz cuts growing out, and some were reveling in having their hair back. A few were clearly struggling with the altitude and one woman had an oxygen tank. But in this group, none of that was exceptional or embarrassing.

"Tell us something unusual about yourself." Beth and Jennifer, the camp directors had us gather in a circle to begin to share and get to know each other.

And the circle began one by one.

"I was born in a taxi."
"My kids think I like the cat better than them – it is a special cat."
"I have made over 300 quilts and give them as prayer quilts to people who are going to the hospital."
"I am a licensed skydiver."
"I am retired Air Force."
"I am a long-distance ocean kayaker."
"I taught elementary school for thirty years."
"I walked the Camino de Santiago in Spain six months after chemo ended."
"I play classical piano."
"I was a fitness coach before cancer and I still am."
"I quit being an accountant after cancer and now I am an artist."
"I am a lawyer."
"I live in New York City but I am a Californian at heart, I am moving to Bodega Bay."
"I married my wife this year."
"I like to shop and wear jewelry — my friends call me Sparkles."
"I am a long-distance cyclist and have cycled through Europe."
"I am writing a musical about ovarian cancer."

And on it went.

Some of these self-descriptions were in the past tense — the person they were and remember from before cancer — the person they hoped to be again in the future. The kayaker who wanted to get back on the ocean. The sky diver now grounded. The Air Force vet on disability. But they knew who they were, just as I did, and they wanted that person back.

Camp also gave us a chance to be vigorous. With ropes, plenty of handhold, and lots of staff assistance – helmets on bald heads and new friends cheering, women old and young scaled the climbing wall. From the 81-year-old former distance cyclist to the woman on hospice care, to the young women in their twenties who were so lovely and should not even be dealing with this disease. Women flew down the zipline with arms out, laughing and screaming. Every morning at 6:30, a small group climbed the butte; the first day they saw a herd of elk passing by. The confidence in their own physical self, which was so damaged by cancer, was buttressed and they laughed as they experienced a new challenge they had not thought they could do.

But beneath it all was our common foe, ovarian cancer. After learning names and where women were from, the next questions were usually about cancer. Anyplace else, with other people who don't share this disease, this would have been unacceptable and rude.

"When were you diagnosed?"
"What stage were you?"
"Where were you treated?"
"Have you had a recurrence?"
"What drugs have you had?"

Julie, the medical oncologist and volunteer camp doctor, and I conducted a round table discussion to answer questions about clinical trials. These trials involve studying the use of new treatments that might work in women with particular tumor characteristics. These trials are for newly diagnosed women as well as those whose initial treatment did not work. Some people say this is for women who "failed" treatment. But I think it is the opposite; it is for women whose treatment "failed" them — or maybe it is best to say it is for women whose treatment was not the perfect fit for their tumor.

Women came to this discussion with questions and confusion. "I have never been told about trials," one said, "why hasn't anyone told me about this? It seems like everyone knows about it but me. My doctor never seems to have the time to explain things to me."

We talked about the procedure for trials, randomization, the need to avoid bias, the care taken to explain the trial and to be sure the required criteria and safety measures are followed. Women most often, learn about trials when they are at the peak of their anxiety, some when they are just diagnosed and some when standard approaches stop working and they have a recurrence. But learning this new information at a peak anxiety level almost guarantees that it will not be well understood.

"I am on my second trial," one said. "They threw me off the first one."

"Why do you think that happened?" I asked.

"Because my markers continued to go up they didn't think it was working."

"And then what happened?" I asked.

"They put me on another trial," she said, "I don't know about this one yet," as she rattles off the complex and seemingly nonsensical names of the drugs.

We talk about NED, our friend NED, otherwise known as "No Evidence of Disease" and how NED came into many lives and then left without saying goodbye when they had a recurrence. With feet dragging, they went back to their PITA friend (pain in the ass) chemo (but a friend nevertheless). We have all wondered if our remissions could become permanent.

The next day I gave a talk about ovarian cancer research. Somehow, despite years of teaching, I was nervous. I had never faced sixty-five women with ovarian cancer before and I wondered if some would ask questions I couldn't answer. And they might not show up at all. They may choose to spend their time in the pool or doing yoga. What if they were all sick and scared, weepy and weak? But it was too late; I volunteered and it was time to put those concerns aside.

Most of the women did show up and they did have lots of questions. When I finished I felt more convinced than ever that women want accurate information just as I had wanted. They want to think about the complexity of the disease, they want to understand the fundamentals of these issues, and they want to understand what is going on with their own bodies.

Women shared stories of being misdiagnosed and of being shuttled between physicians who saw symptoms that looked like gastrointestinal bloating and discomfort but were in fact common ovarian cancer symptoms. There were young women who were told they were too young to get ovarian cancer and old women who were told their symptoms were just old age; both old and young were disregarded. Some were angry after being treated by physicians who they later suspected were not experts in ovarian cancer and did not refer them until they faced a recurrence. I was again confronted with the realization that my own experience was not typical. I was treated at my place of work by people I had known for decades, and after a Stage IV diagnosis, I continued in remission.

A psychologist, Vivien, has volunteered year after year at the camp to help bring calm. She has what she calls a "toolbox of strategies" that she shared to address the challenges of fear and negotiation. "There are ways to not get overwhelmed, deal with one issue at a time, maintain control, and to know when to put away the constant worry and choose to do something in opposition to the fear."

She helped us learn that it is OK to sort through our friendships and find those friends who are supportive, nurture those with bigger hearts and to let others go. We shared the crazy and insensitive statements that people make.

One woman said someone told her she was a "goner".

Someone told another woman, "Everyone I know with that disease is dead".

Another said that a sister-in-law said, "My friends are dropping like flies and now you too." It is never good to be compared to a fly.

Another told the story of friends and family who never called and never asked how she was. One told of a husband that just left. What do you say when the worst response comes from family?

And juxtaposed against all of these, were the wonderful families, the giving friends and the extraordinary clinicians who supported them through this hard time. We ended with tears when one woman told her story. When her hair fell out and she asked her sister to shave her head; surrounded by her mother and her three sisters, one-by-one, they all shaved their heads in solidarity.

Many had children at home, adolescent and preadolescent children still needing to be raised and nurtured by a mother who was distracted by her own disease and afraid that those children might grow up without her. Some children stepped up while others distanced themselves emotionally. Some women were still hiding the seriousness of the illness from their kids, or at least hiding their fear of it. They sent their children off to school and then worried during the day even as they tried to continue working and managing the household.

And maybe because powerlessness was a common reaction, turning to God was a common response. Not all, but many women turned to faith in a higher power and reentered a calm state by letting the future rest in that higher power however they understood it. "Face the treatment, just do it — leave the rest up to God." I heard this more than any other way of living with cancer.

In the art workshop, I asked the women to think of the words that helped them get through their diagnosis and treatment or the words they wanted to say to the people who helped them get through.

"Cancer and treatment can take away your voice, your ability to express how you feel, to ask your questions. All of us can feel powerless and afraid. Think about what words you said to yourself to get you through. It can be a word like "hope". It can be scripture like the psalms or the beatitudes. It can be a quote from a person like Gandhi. It can be simple like, 'I will be well.' My words were 'Gratitude, Integrity and Determination' and when I began to lose myself, these words helped me find myself again."

There was no hesitation as women quickly wrote out their words.
"Braveheart"
"Buoyant"
"Be fit be awesome"
"God is with me"
"You are the wind beneath my wings"
"I am loved"
"Faith"

I showed them ways they could use their words in their art and shared the work of Sister Corita Kent and others to provide examples. And then, using collage, cut paper, writing, and paint they incorporated their words into their art.

A day later a beautiful young woman, showed me the bird she created with tissue paper collage and the words that inspired her "I will not let this steal my joy."
"It is beautiful. You need to frame it," I told her.
"I will," she said, "it will go over my bed."

The last night we sang folk songs and show tunes. We swam in the pool and sat in the hot tub one last time. Too quickly it was time to leave. We exchanged information and promised to stay in touch at least on Facebook.

I returned to camp in 2018 and 2019. I saw some of the same women and friendships continued on and became stronger. Maybe I will see some of the same women next year and the year after. But some did not return. Sadly, some of these vibrant and courageous women died from their disease — all before their time.

Chapter 35: Step Up

What do cancer advocates do? They speak for the living, they speak for the ill, they speak for our children, and they speak for those who have died.

When I was first diagnosed and on chemo, I met another woman, an eight-year survivor. "You are a long-term survivor," I said, feeling immediately encouraged.

"Yes, but it always comes back," she adamantly replied. "I have been on several treatments, I'm now on a clinical trial, but it will come back." She warned me to expect a recurrence. And here I was just starting treatment. I really was not ready to talk about a recurrence. I avoided talking with her after that conversation and I avoided support groups because I did not want to be discouraged by such stories while I was getting through treatment and just needing to focus on myself. But also, I had friends who had gone through cancer treatment and some still on chemotherapy, so they were my support group.

Although time has passed, my fear can still be reignited as others reveal their recurring disease and need to gather themselves to again face whatever treatment they must undergo next. The recurrences among those who have gone a long time with no evidence of disease are like matches to the waiting dry leaves of fear that hang on me and can easily be reignited.

One of my students leant me the Lance Armstrong book, *It's Not About the Bike,* the story of his survival of late-stage testicular cancer with metastases to his lungs and brain. I bought a *Live Strong* t-shirt from his foundation that I still wear. His story told me it was possible to survive even the worst cancer. While his image was tarnished later by his use of performance drugs, his recovery, his athletic accomplishments, and his perseverance told me that there could be life after cancer. For a survivor of metastatic cancer to even think about entering the Tour De France was almost a superhero fantasy to me.

Now, I want to be the survivor against the odds that might give hope to other women with ovarian cancer. I want to hear their stories and to learn from their experience and I want to tell them my story. I am on a Facebook community of women with ovarian cancer from all over the country and no two stories seem the same. Some are ill with what seems to be uncontrollable and unrelenting disease, side effects, bowel blockages, and exhaustion. And there are women sending messages of encouragement to each other. Ovarian cancer is somewhat rare and can feel isolating; the Facebook community provides a means of support.

I know women like me who have survived late-stage ovarian cancer. And every day I read of women traveling, loving, working, and making a difference in their own way. I want to say to the newly diagnosed women, "you don't know what will happen, you need to do your best with the treatment, and live on. It can be treated and it doesn't always come back." Sometimes I wonder if this helps or hurts. There is always the question of why some get lucky and others do not, and if you are in the "not" group do you really want to hear from the "lucky" group? But like me, I imagine that those newly diagnosed want to hear about the possibility that they can get better. It is called "beating cancer" like it is some sort of athletic competition. But, if I wanted to hear about Lance Armstrong, and his testicular cancer, then maybe other people with ovarian or other cancers would want to hear my story to give them strength and hope.

I have heard the expression "survivor guilt" applied to those in war who survive while their friends are killed. President George H.W. Bush was said to have thought every day of his crewmates who died when his airplane was shot down in the Pacific in World War II and he ejected safely and was picked up. Such experiences can be met with depression, with moving on and forgetting, or with giving back in some way, to try to make up for those who were tragically lost. Those who inexplicably survive can often not help but revisit and ask "why?" even though there are no answers. According to Bush's friends, survivor guilt spurred him toward service to country for the rest of his life. This was his way of paying-up for the lives lost.

I always planned that when I retired I would leave cancer and AIDS behind me. I would do something of service, perhaps tutoring children, or teaching art to children who had no art class in their schools. Maybe I would raise seeing-eye puppies or search and rescue dogs. Maybe I would become a volunteer forest ranger. But more cancer work? No, that was not in the cards for me.

Despite these plans, by the time I retired from my job conducting cancer and AIDS research, I had survived Stage IV ovarian cancer. I knew that I could not just walk away and ignore it. I could not say, "well, I am well now so I just want to move on like it never happened." It did happen. I felt that terror. I went through those 16 months of infusions and surgery and the follow-on years of watching and waiting.

Now, rather than resenting being pulled back into the cancer world during my retirement, I see it as an opportunity to use what I know both as a scientist and as a cancer survivor to help other women. I don't have survivor guilt. Instead, I have survivor gratitude and that, as well as my own continuing curiosity about the biology of cancer, has led me to become an advocate for research and education of women with ovarian cancer. If I were not doing this I would feel guilty, not for surviving but for not helping. Walking away would have diminished me and negligent guilt rather than survivor guilt would have hung on me.

The opportunities to conduct advocacy on any illness are many, and that is particularly true for ovarian cancer. Ovarian cancer has received less attention and less funding than would be justified on the basis of lives lost in comparison with other diseases such as breast and prostate cancer. The incidence is lower for ovarian cancer but the mortality rate is much higher. The lack of attention means that women with this disease are experiencing slower development of drugs tailored to the idiosyncrasy of ovarian cancer cells.

Through the Ovarian Cancer Research Alliance (OCRA) I have advocated for additional funding for ovarian cancer research. OCRA coordinates visits by survivors and family members, with Senators and Congressmen/women. In March 2019, I visited four senators and three representatives to tell them about the disease and the need for research dollars. Six of these signed on to the congressional letters to increase funding specifically for ovarian cancer research and this effort increased ovarian cancer funding by 15 million dollars.

I participate as a speaker for the OCRA Survivors Teaching Students (STS) program. This program provides speakers to tell their stories of detection, treatment, and survival after diagnosis to medical and nursing students in training, who know surprisingly little about this disease and have many questions. We stress the subtle symptoms of this cancer. We also stress the need for referral to gynecologic oncologists who specialize in this disease. But perhaps the most important message is simply the power of our presence.

I volunteer at Camp Mak-A-Dream in Gold Creek Montana in the fall. It is at this camp that I have learned the most about the individual experiences women have with this disease and have developed friendships with other women with ovarian cancer. And it is this camp that has fueled my energy as well as my sorrow as I hear the stories of women who attend and mourn those who die.

*

My greatest satisfaction comes from being a patient advocate on research studies. In 2015, my colleagues Drs. Malcolm Pike and Leigh Pearce applied for a research grant called the Multidisciplinary Ovarian Cancer Outcomes Group (MOCOG). I had just retired and they asked me to be a patient advocate on this study that involves investigators from Canada, England, Australia, and the US. The study investigates immunologic, genetic, clinical, and lifestyle factors in order to understand the important predictors of long-term survival (of 10 years or more) for women who have Stage III or IV high grade serous ovarian cancer (the most common cell type) as compared to those who survive for a shorter period of time with the same stage of disease. Part of the purpose of being a patient advocate on this research study is to communicate the information I learn to other women with the disease.

Three other patient advocates were also invited to participate in MOCOG. Bronwyn is from Australia and is a young mother who also has earned a PhD in Chemistry. Cindy is active with FORCE, and organization for women who are at familial risk for ovarian cancer. Anne is from Canada and works in every way and every day to raise funds, to organize support groups, and to address members of Canadian parliament. Each of us takes the information we learn and uses it to educate other women and support women who have developed this disease. Each of us also advocates for funding. Each of us talks with the researchers to help them understand this disease from our perspective, to speak for women with ovarian cancer. And each of us proves there is life after ovarian cancer.

The MOCOG study is a step to try to make such progress for ovarian cancer with the objective of understanding the immunologic, genetic and lifestyle factors that are important for ovarian cancer survival. Not surprisingly, the immune system is very important to fighting cancer but it seems that the tumor itself has the ability to block the immune defenses. This leads to investigations of how to overcome this blocking and develop new therapies that will allow the immune system to destroy the tumor. In addition, genetic mutations that are inherited or that occur only inside the tumor itself can lead to longer or shorter survival. At some time in the future the perfect match between the genetic mutations in the tumor and the particular chemo or immune therapies that will kill those tumor cells will become known. Scientists have already made such progress with some other cancers.

The lifestyle factors have been extensively examined with regard to risk of developing this disease. But fewer studies have looked at whether those risk factors have an impact on survival after the disease develops. In addition to finding experts to provide care and complying with treatment regimens, women need information on how to help themselves after diagnosis, and the studies are looking at those issues as well. All women want to be able to do something to regain their health and kill the cancer, but there is very little scientific information to tell women what to do. In the absence of that, women do the best they can. But some are susceptible to unproven, expensive, and ineffective "potions." It is imperative that the lifestyle questions like diet and exercise, be answered. There are epidemiologic studies suggesting that common drugs such as aspirin and statins given after diagnosis will also improve survival. As advocates, we seek to encourage clinical trials on these findings. Clinical trials are the only way to verify and test the epidemiologic findings.

*

But these are not the only issues for advocates such as myself. One of the major messages of advocacy groups is to assure that women are effectively treated. According to a research report (Cochrane Collaboration report), women treated for ovarian cancer at comprehensive cancer centers had higher survival rates. The expertise of the doctors and nurses that provide the treatment make a huge difference. Removing all visible tumor during surgery is a major indicator of survival. Only surgeons who perform this surgery regularly can develop the highest level of expertise to conduct this complex and lengthy surgery. It only stands to reason that this would be true. It is also the people that patients don't see, the technicians doing the scans, the radiologist who reads them, the phlebotomist who takes the blood and the lab technician who analyzes it, the nurse who infuses the chemo but also the pharmacist who mixes it – everyone needs to get it right. It is a well-trained team. But sadly, not all women are referred and sometimes non-experts wrongly believe they can treat this disease effectively and they only refer when the disease recurs. Many women with ovarian cancer are not treated according to approved protocols. This means that some women who are not treated effectively at the start will have a reduced chance of survival.

We need centers-of-excellence for ovarian cancer, places where the nearly 23,000 women diagnosed with this disease every year in the US can get optimal care. I know this is possible because it was achieved for pediatric cancers that are almost exclusively treated at specialty hospitals. No non-expert community pediatrician would treat a child with cancer. While children with cancer are referred to centers of excellence, that is not the case for ovarian cancer. But it should be. Even now, with what is already know, survival rates could be improved if every woman was seen at a center of excellence for ovarian cancer. Furthermore, at research centers, tumor tissue is frozen, banked, saved, and studied. Questionnaires are answered, and clinical trials are completed. Knowledge grows. Not only do patients get better care but they also contribute to research and knowledge, and that is a gift.

Furthermore, survival times for cancer patients who are poor is shorter. The issues of insurance coverage, access to expert medical care, education about the disease, work demands, and a myriad of other interferences with care in low-income communities are important advocacy issues. Many women may experience delays or be covered under systems that are a "take what you can get" variety and not optimal. As a student at the UCLA School of Public Health in 1970, I first heard the mantra "health care is a right not a privilege." Now 50 years later, that mantra is still being repeated and "healthcare for all" still has not happened. It is unconscionable and it is something that can and should be changed.

In the past 50 years there have been many breakthroughs in cancer therapy that have made many cancers curable. There were breakthroughs in pediatric leukemia therapy that turned it all around — that made it a curable disease and not a death sentence. And I saw first-hand when this happened for HIV/AIDS when the new drugs, protease inhibitors, were developed in 1996 and caused the death rate to plunge. This is beginning to happen now for ovarian cancer. Bevacizumab was approved in 2014 for ovarian cancer and is now being used in combination with other drugs. New therapies like PARP Inhibitors for ovarian cancer are available now and these are being used in combination with the older chemotherapies. These drugs were not even developed or approved ten years ago when I was diagnosed. Progress is being made.

Chapter 36: Back to Normal

It has been ten years since I was diagnosed.

People ask if I feel back to "normal."

"Oh yes," I say. "I am ten years older, but I think I feel about how I would if I had not had cancer at all, if I had not gone through those 16 months of treatment, if my hair had not fallen out and my stomach had not felt like it turned inside out. Except for the tinnitus, I think my body has recovered. The resilience of the human body is amazing."

But a part of me dawdles and hangs back in those dark days. There is a drain on my mind needing to keep insisting on resilience. It is natural, my mind wants to recover just as my body did. I now plan for the future. I bought a new car without worrying that I shouldn't do that, and I got the crown put on my tooth.

To some extent it is hard to remember the fear, except that the fear never completely leaves. I know I am never completely safe. I need to remind myself that nobody is completely safe from everything. Now I live with the ease of the recovered and every year it does not come back is another increment of ease I feel, another increment of putting the cancer behind me, and living with my present good health.

After treatment ended and people would ask how I was doing – I would always say "fine." On good days and bad days, my answer was the same. But it was unsatisfying to me. "Fine" is not the right word. At some point I switched to the word "well." When the cashier at Trader Joes asks, "How are you doing today?" I say, "I am well thank you." I say it to myself, "I am well." And I remember the nurse who did my scans who told me that when she had breast cancer she would hug herself and say "I will be well." And then I say to myself and everyone else who asks whether in the casual passing or the close friendship, "I am well" and in saying this out loud I am affirming it for myself.

A few months ago, after going in for my annual follow-up visit, I told a friend that everything still looked good, no sign of recurrence. She looked surprised. "Are you still getting checked for that?" she asked.

I had not realized I not told her of my checkups. "Yes, of course," I said.

"How long will you have to do that?" she asked.

"I don't know, maybe the rest of my life. I haven't really thought about ending."

And that's it. It does not end. It is there even though it fades. I changed in that I now understand I am vulnerable. I know some wayward cell could start this or something else all over again and I won't even feel it until it has crept to places in my body far from where it started. I may not live with fear as I did at first, but I do live with a sense of vulnerability. I live with a distrust of my body that was never there until the day I was diagnosed but also I live with the trust of my body to recover. The feelings are sometimes in opposition but yet both are held in my mind simultaneously. And I live with the knowledge that life is not guaranteed and is hopelessly short and still I can waste much of it on foolishness even after I have had the wake-up call that it could all end without warning. But if you ask me how I am – I will tell you, "I am well," and I believe that is now true.

Chapter 37: Back to Zion National Park

In 2018 and 2019, I returned to Camp Mak-A-Dream in Montana. Many women who I had first met in 2017 returned and we renewed our friendships. But as I feared, many did not return. Many of the stunning women who shared their stories with me had died, and it is in their names that I continue to advocate for ovarian cancer research.

In the silent auction at camp in 2019, I bought a turquoise necklace that was donated by a young woman diagnosed with ovarian cancer in her twenties. When I first met her I thought she could not have this disease and must be there with a family member. But unfortunately, she was the one with this disease and that realization shook and angered me at this injustice.

This necklace is my talisman. It reminds me how much work is left to be done. I wore this necklace when I went to visit four members of the Senate and three members of the House of Representatives to ask them to please support more funding for ovarian cancer research. But mostly it reminds me of the young woman who donated it to the auction, who developed this disease at such a young age, who approached the challenges of ovarian cancer with resilience, determination, and faith, who hiked and loved her husband and her dogs, who traveled despite the recurrences, and who said she would not let this disease steal her joy. She deserved better. She inspires me.

In April 2019, I traveled back to Zion National Park as an advocate along with Anne, Cindy, and Bronwyn to the annual meetings of the Ovarian Cancer Association Consortium (OCAC) and the MOCOG study. We met at the Las Vegas airport where I rented an SUV, and we made the 160-mile road trip to Zion talking and laughing the entire way.

Zion National Park is where my story began with the increasing fatigue I felt on our way to Yellowstone in the summer of 2010, two weeks before I was diagnosed. The thyroid scan and the needle biopsy of the node in my neck that showed ovarian cancer, were still two weeks away. Unbeknownst to me, cancer was spreading throughout my body. But I was ignorant to it. I was in the naïve days before this entire story began to unfold.

As I walked the trails in the canyon again in 2019, I marveled at the beauty just as I had in 2010. Zion is known for the red rock canyon walls with the river running through the middle and a few recently released California condors flying overhead. Deer wandered the canyon floor unafraid of the tourists, and wild turkeys flaunted their tail feathers. As I walked some of the same lower trails of Zion Canyon I thought about the years that had passed. Now I am a long-term survivor and an exceptional responder. But I clearly remember the shock of the cancer diagnosis and the demands of the chemo and surgery that followed.

At the meetings we listened to geneticists, immunologists, epidemiologists, and clinicians who are dedicated to studying this disease. It is our responsibility to give them feedback, to stretch our understanding of the technical research, and to take what we learn home and make it understandable to other women with the disease. It is our responsibility to advocate for additional funding. And it is up to us to thank them for the work they are doing.

"Keep working," "try harder" I whisper to myself as I think about the researchers I am working with. "Keep at it – the answers will come."

And when the answers come, women around the world will benefit. Ovarian cancer will be curable, and we will all rejoice.

APPENDIX

Jean LeCerf Richardson

MORE INFORMATION FOR WOMEN WITH OVARIAN CANCER

While massive campaigns have helped women learn about breast cancer, the same cannot be said about ovarian cancer. This appendix will provide some basic information taken from expert sources. While it is not meant to be a medical resource, it may help women understand more so that they can be informed about their own disease, ask questions, and be involved in their own care. It will provide a base for understanding what the common terms are in managing ovarian cancer and understanding these terms will help communication with health care providers. There are many good sources to learn more about ovarian cancer and some are listed here.

Where you can find more information.

There are many sources of excellent information on the internet and there are probably even more sources of erroneous information. Please avoid the many sites that will try to sell you potions and notions that are inaccurate and will take your money and time and interfere with quality medical care. The resources listed here are reputable and the information can be trusted.

National Institutes of Health: National Cancer Institute:
www.cancer.gov
The NCI website is an excellent source of information about symptoms, screening, statistics, staging, and treatment including NCI supported clinical trials. NCI recognized Comprehensive Cancer Centers are listed and offer expert cancer treatment.

www.clinicaltrials.gov This is where you can look for clinical trials. This is an exhaustive list of thousands of clinical trials so it takes searching to determine what might be appropriate. Because there are so many caveats about who can be admitted to a trial in terms of stage, other health conditions, prior treatment, and so forth, it is difficult for the average person to wade through this and you might need help from your doctor or nurse.

Ovarian Cancer Research Alliance: www.ocrahope.org
The Ovarian Cancer Research Alliance supports advocacy and research. The OCRA National Conference held in July each year is a good place to meet other women with ovarian cancer and to hear excellent presentations of current research. The conference is held in alternating years between Washington DC and cities across the country.

FORCE (Facing Our Risk of Cancer Empowered)
www.facingourrisk.org This organization provides education and advocacy for those with genetic risk for breast, ovarian and related cancers.

American Cancer Society: www.cancer.org
The American Cancer Society is the largest non-governmental organization addressing the needs of cancer patients as well as the funding for cancer research. The website provides search options for various services you may need including medical, social services, financial, advocacy, support groups etc.

Two excellent recent journal publications and a book:

National Academies of Sciences, Engineering and Medicine 2016. *Ovarian Cancers: Evolving Paradigms in Research and Care*. Institute of Medicine: Washington DC The National Academies Press. This is available online.

Hematology / Oncology Clinics of North America December 32(6), 2018
Ursula A Matulonis, MD Editor
A good source for recent scientific reviews of ovarian cancer. The entire December 2018 publication is devoted to ovarian cancer reviews including the most common type, High Grade Serous, and the less common types such as Low Grade and Clear Cell. It also addresses treatment and recurrence issues.

Bristow,RE., Cornelison, TL., & Montz, FJ. eds *A Guide to Survivorship for Women Who Have Ovarian Cancer (second edition)*. Baltimore MD: Johns Hopkins University Press, 2015. This is a good resource in general. But because some of the newer treatments came out after this book was published, it will not be a good resource for the most recent advances in new drugs such as PARP Inhibitors.

Resources for Treatment: Finding the best places to receive treatment for ovarian cancer is very important – both to locate an experienced gynecological oncology surgeon as well as an experienced gynecological oncologist or medical oncologist who handles chemotherapy. In many cancer centers, the surgeon also handles the chemotherapy. Research is going on all over the country, but especially at NCI designated Comprehensive Cancer Centers. So that is a good place to start your search and these are listed on the NCI website.

How common is Ovarian Cancer and what do we know about survival?[1,2]

According to the NCI, in 2016 there were an estimated 15,338,988 people living with cancer of any type in the United States, and of these 229,875 were living with ovarian cancer. Some of these women would be in treatment for initial disease or recurrences, some would be in remission, and some would be long-term survivors.

Cancer is not an uncommon disease, but ovarian cancer is considered rare. In 2019 in the United States, 1,762,450 people will be diagnosed with cancer and 606,880 will die from cancer. Of these, approximately 23,000 women will get ovarian cancer and 14,000 will die from it in 2019. That means one in every 78 women will get it. Many women will not know any other woman who has had this disease.

In contrast, breast cancer will account for 268,600 new cases in 2019, and 41,760 women will die from it. One in eight women will get this disease. I suspect every woman knows someone who has had breast cancer.

But the outlook for cancer varies greatly. Sixty seven percent of people with any cancer survive five years as compared with 90% of women with breast cancer and 48% of women with ovarian cancer. While the occurrence of ovarian cancer is less common than breast cancer the risk of dying once it is diagnosed, is higher.

So, what is the importance of these numbers?

As defined by the National Cancer Institute, cancers that occur in fewer than 15 out of 100,000 people each year are considered **rare** cancers. Ovarian cancer occurs in 11.4 women in every 100,000 each year, so that makes ovarian cancer rare. Rare cancers are often more difficult to prevent, diagnose and treat than the more common cancers. And because there are fewer of them, research is more difficult and less money is spent to address them.

There is good news and bad news about ovarian cancer.

---

[1] SEER Cancer Stat Facts. National Cancer Institute, Bethesda MD

[2] These data will change as the years go by but updated information is readily available on the NCI website.

First, the good news. The number of new cases of ovarian cancer has gone down. While 25 years ago there were over 14 new cases per 100,000 women, now there are 11.4 cases as already noted above. So, if it was rare before, it is even rarer now. This is likely due to three reasons. First, women who have used birth control pills for five years or more are less likely to get this disease, and use of birth control pills is more common now. Second, women who breastfed their babies are also less likely to get this disease and there has been an increase in breastfeeding. And finally, as information has increased about genetic risk due to inheriting the BRCA1 or BRCA2 mutation, many women with these mutations have responded by having preventive surgery thus decreasing their risk. More about this later.

But now the bad news. In terms of five-year survival rates after diagnosis, according to the National Cancer Institute the all-cancer survival rate increased from 49% in 1975 to 70% in 2011. For breast cancer the increase is 75% to 91%; and for ovarian cancer the increase is 34% to 49% over the same time period. While there has clearly been an improvement in five-year survival, still there is work to be done. But it should be noted that these data may improve as the new PARP inhibitors are introduced to widespread use. It will take more time to fully evaluate the impact of these new drugs in terms of five-year survival rates.

Finally, it is worth noting that this disease is worldwide. Globally, 240,000 women are diagnosed with ovarian cancer every year and it will cause 150,000 deaths. [3] Researchers around the world are studying ovarian cancer and when progress is made it helps women worldwide.[4]

---

[3] Ferlay, J. Soerjomataram I, Ervik M et al GLPBPCAM 2012 v1.0 Cancer Incidence and Mortality Worldwide: IARC Cancer base No.

[4] Lyon France, International Agency for Research on Cancer: 2013. http://globocan.iarc.fr

Who gets ovarian cancer?[5]

As with most cancer types, ovarian cancer increases with age. Ovarian cancer is most frequently diagnosed between the ages of 55 and 64. The median age at diagnosis is 63 which means that half of the cases occur among those younger than 63 and half in those over the age of 63. This is about the same age as for breast cancer. For cancers overall, the median age is 72. So, from that perspective, both ovarian and breast cancers skew toward the younger side. While we don't often think about cancer among young adults, for ovarian cancer 5.3% of patients are under age 35. This means it is affecting them just as they may be starting families.

In terms of ethnicity, ovarian cancer is most common among White women followed in order, by Hispanic women, Black women, Asian women, and Native American women.

[5] SEER Cancer Stat Facts, National Cancer Institute, Bethesda, MD

What Are the Symptoms of Ovarian Cancer?

One of the major obstacles to improved survival of ovarian cancer is that it is most often diagnosed late, at stage III or IV. Why does this occur?

There are several reasons for this. First, the ovaries are deep inside the abdomen and it is difficult to feel what might be going on with them. Whereas a lump in the breast might be noticed rather quickly by a woman, a lump on the ovaries will not be noticed. Also, the ovaries don't have an opening that is accessible as does, the mouth, the throat, the cervix and the colon. The opening or surface of the colon, for example, is accessible and can be examined with a scope during a colonoscopy and any precancerous polyps can be removed. Similarly, cells on the opening or surface of the cervix can be scraped off during a pap smear and looked at under the microscope. The surface of the ovary or the fallopian tubes cannot be seen with a scope or tested by means of a pap smear. Finally, bleeding can be a sign of colon cancer, uterine cancer and some other cancers, but rarely for ovarian cancer. And there is no blood test or other screening test for ovarian cancer – an issue that will be dealt with below. So how would a woman suspect that she has this disease at an early stage?

Ovarian cancer is not completely silent but it certainly only whispers and the symptoms are so non-specific that they may appear to be indigestion, irritable bowel, or some other stomach or intestinal problem. And because ovarian cancer diagnosis increases with age the symptoms can be ignored as a sign of aging or even the complaints of the "worried well." Nevertheless, the symptoms that whisper have been identified and these subtle symptoms, when they appear, can lead to diagnosis and treatment.

Most websites provide a list of common symptoms. Memorial Sloan Kettering Cancer Center in New York City lists the following symptoms of ovarian cancer:

- abdominal bloating or swelling
- pain in the abdomen or pelvis
- difficulty eating, or feeling full quickly
- lack of appetite
- feeling an urgent need to urinate
- needing to urinate frequently
- change in bowel habits (constipation or diarrhea)
- change in menstrual periods

- vaginal bleeding between periods
- back pain
- weight gain or loss

To this list, I would add my symptom of fatigue. It may be that I felt this symptom because the cancer had already spread to my lymphatic system, which of course means it was already advanced stage. These vague symptoms can be missed easily. Most often women end up going to their general practitioner and may even get referred to a gastrointestinal specialist. When these symptoms are present, ovarian cancer needs to be on the list of possibilities. These symptoms may be consistent over a period of time and may alert women to notice that something has changed and they don't feel "normal." As the symptoms progress and become more severe, the urgency to reach a diagnosis increases, more tests are run and eventually the diagnosis is reached. But precious time may be lost and the cancer may spread. That lost time means treatment is delayed and the disease becomes more difficult to treat effectively. As with all cancers, early diagnosis is one of the keys to survival.

What are the types of ovarian cancer?[6]

There are several different types of ovarian tumors that differ depending upon the cells that give rise to the tumor. Epithelial cell ovarian cancers are the most common. These are divided into five types: High Grade Serous is the most common epithelial tumor, followed by Clear Cell, Endometroid, Mucinous and Low Grade Serous. These different types of epithelial cancers are characterized by different mutations in the tumor cells and they look different under the microscope. In addition, epithelial cancers include some that are considered transitional or undifferentiated and don't fit into one of the previous categories.

In addition to these subtypes of epithelial ovarian cancers, there are a small number of sex cord stromal cell tumors including granulosa cell tumors. And there are also a small number of germ cell ovarian tumors.

These different types of ovarian cancers are identified by examination of cells from the tumor under the microscope by a highly trained pathologist. The treatment for each of these may vary and this is why it is very important that the specific type is correctly identified. As research progresses it is increasingly possible to target the treatment to the specific ovarian cancer cell subtype.

When pathologists look at the tumor cells under the microscope, they will also assign a grade to the cells. Tumor cells are cells that have mutations and abnormal changes. Grading is a way of assessing how abnormal the cells look in comparison to normal ovarian cells. If the cells are Grade 1, they look almost like healthy cells. You may hear this called "well-differentiated" or "low grade." As the abnormalities increase, the grade increases as well. Grade 3 tumors are very abnormal and no longer look like ovarian cells. These are called " poorly differentiated" tumors. The grade as well as the stage are important factors in determining treatment and prognosis.

What are some of the risk factors for ovarian cancer?[7,8]

---

[6] Ovarian Cancer Research Alliance: www.ocrahope.org

[7] Ovarian Cancer Research Alliance: www.ocrahope.org

[8] Webb, PM, and Jordan SJ. Epidemiology of Epithelial Ovarian Cancer. Best Practice and Research Clinical Obstetrics and Gynecology v.41, May 2017, pages 3-14.

Epidemiologists have identified several factors that either increase or decrease the risk of developing ovarian cancer. While this may not seem very helpful for women who already have the disease, it is tremendously important in the effort to decrease the occurrence of the disease in the future. A further note is that while the information provided here is for ovarian cancer rates overall, some of these may differ for the less common subtypes of ovarian cancer.

Ovarian cancer, like breast cancer, is related to hormonal factors and this is manifest in its relationship with childbearing, breastfeeding, use of oral contraceptives, and menopausal hormones. However, some factors have received strong and consistent confirmation while other results have been inconsistent.

Factors that decrease risk:

Removal of the ovaries and/or the fallopian tubes

Women who have given birth are at 10-20 percent reduced risk for each birth.

Women who have given birth and breast feed their babies have a reduced risk by 20-25%.

The use of combined oral contraceptive pills is protective against developing ovarian cancer. There is approximately a 20% reduction of risk for every five years of use.

Tubal ligation has been shown to be associated with a 20-30% reduced risk of ovarian cancer.

Use of anti-inflammatory medication (aspirin, NSAIDS) and increased physical activity has been associated with a reduced risk of ovarian cancer.

Factors that increase risk:

Family history of breast, ovarian, uterine, or colorectal cancer in a grandmother, mother, daughter, or sister. Don't ignore family history that is paternal such as your paternal grandmother or aunts.

Mutations in BRCA1 or BRCA2 genes and related genes (RAD51C, RAD 51D, BRIP1, PALB2) or Lynch syndrome

Early menarche and late menopause have been associated with increased risk.

A diagnosis of endometriosis has been associated with a two-to-three-fold increased risk of ovarian cancer primarily for endometroid and clear cell ovarian cancer.

Increased risk has been associated with obesity and with sedentary lifestyle.

Unknown risk or needs more study:

Studies of hormone replacement therapy at menopause has resulted in conflicting results and may relate to the exact hormone mix used. This needs further study.

Alcohol use, coffee or tea drinking, and diet have not been shown to be associated with ovarian cancer risk.

Another controversy concerns the use of talcum powder in the genital area but the research is mixed with regard to this particular issue.

Summary:

Taken together, these findings indicate that ovarian cancer is a disease that is related to natural hormone changes and with hormonal preparations. This is one of the most robust findings with regard to risk elevation or reduction. Exactly how this might work with regard to biological mechanisms is uncertain. The strongest protective factors (oral contraceptives, pregnancy, breast feeding) all inhibit ovulation and this may reduce the occurrence of mutations related to inflammation and cellular repair. Findings on risk factors for ovarian cancer continue to emerge. As factors are confirmed in multiple studies, confidence in these results strengthens.

What does it mean to be at Genetic Risk? [9]

All people inherit BRCA1 and BRCA2 genes from their parents. These genes are important for DNA repair to protect the cell from genetic damage. In some cases, these genes are mutated and that mutation can also be inherited. BRCA mutations increase the risk for breast and ovarian cancers. If the BRCA genes are mutated, they cannot perform the function of DNA repair and cells may develop additional mutations that can lead to cancer. BRCA gene mutations are present in about 1 in 400 people but this varies by ethnic group. These mutations are more common among women with ethnic origins from India or women with Ashkenazi Jewish origins, although women of any ethnicity can carry these mutations.

According to the NCI, [10] approximately 1.3% of all women will develop ovarian cancer; but 44% of women who inherit a BRCA1 mutation and 17% of women who inherit a BRCA2 mutation will develop ovarian cancer by age 80. Inherited mutations are associated with approximately 10-25% of ovarian cancer cases depending on the subtype. Similarly, 12% of all women develop breast cancer in their lifetime; but 72% of women who inherit a BRCA1 mutation and 69% of women who inherit a BRCA2 mutation will develop breast cancer by age 80.

The consequence of this information is twofold. 1)Not all women with these mutations will develop cancer but the risk is very high. 2) Only some women who develop ovarian cancer will have these mutations so for most women with ovarian cancer, these mutations will not be present.

This has led to the following recommendations:

1. Women who have ovarian cancer should be tested for BRCA gene mutations and other mutations that confer greater risk. This is now a standard recommendation for all women who have ovarian cancer.

There are two very important reasons for this.

---

[9] FORCE www.facingourrisk.org

[10] National Cancer Institute. www.cancer.gov

First, women with BRCA1 and BRCA2 mutations will likely be prescribed PARP inhibitors. While women without these mutations may also be placed on PARP inhibitors, women with these mutations seem to benefit the most from PARP inhibitors.

Second, women who have BRCA1 and BRCA2 mutations are likely to have other relatives with these mutations who may be at risk of developing ovarian or breast cancer. These can be daughters, nieces, and sisters. Women found to have a BRCA mutation, are encouraged to share that information with these relatives so that they can get tested and receive counseling about their options to address this risk. In many cases this will include some form of preventive surgery. These are delicate and anxiety producing conversations that should be part of the genetic counseling. While these are difficult conversations in a family, I also am convinced they are easier conversations than a new cancer diagnosis.

2. Women who are healthy but have a family history of ovarian cancer should be tested for these gene mutations. This is true for women with a family history, even if the woman who had the disease has not been tested or is no longer alive. Women can inherit these genes from their mother or father so this includes maternal as well as paternal blood relatives with ovarian cancer.

3. If the test results show a BRCA1/2 mutation, expert help should be obtained from a genetic counselor in making decisions about how to manage this elevated risk. First and foremost, it is important to learn about the options that might include preventive surgery or surveillance. This will depend on your desire to have more children, your age, the specific mutation, other circumstances and your preferences.

4. Women with Ashkenazi Jewish ancestry are more likely to carry mutations in the BRCA1 or BRCA2 genes that confer greater risk (1 in 40) and should be tested for these mutations.

There is another additional consideration that you should be aware of. In most cases BRCA1 and BRCA2 mutations are inherited – they pass from parent to child and are carried in every body cell. However, the ovarian cancer tumor itself develops mutations that are found only in the tumor. These mutations can include BRCA1 and BRCA2. For this reason, more and more cancer centers offer <u>tumor testing</u> to find BRCA1 and BRCA2 mutations in the tumor. This is done to determine the correct treatment for the ovarian cancer tumor itself.

How is Ovarian Cancer Diagnosed?[11]

A number of tests are required to reach a diagnosis. In general, the steps include a 1) medical history and physical exam, 2) blood tests, 3) imaging scans and 4) biopsy.

1) Medical history and physical exam

Family history is a very important component of diagnosis. A strong family history of breast or ovarian cancer suggests an elevated risk of ovarian cancer although many women will not have such a history. In addition, the physician will ask about symptoms and their intensity, duration, and timing. During the physical exam the physician will do a pelvic exam to check for an enlarged ovary or fluid in the abdomen as well as any enlarged lymph nodes.

2) Blood tests

The CA-125 test measures the level of a protein that is frequently produced by ovarian cancer cells. It is not used as a screening test because sometimes it is elevated when women do not have ovarian cancer and not elevated when they do have it. However, because it is usually elevated in women with ovarian cancer it provides additional information to help reach a diagnosis. The CA-125 test is also often used to monitor the response to a course of chemotherapy treatment as well.

3) Imaging

A transvaginal ultrasound is used to provide an image of the ovaries to see if they look enlarged and to see if it looks like there is a tumor or mass on them. The physician will insert a small probe into the woman's vagina that gives off sound waves. A gel substance is placed on the woman's abdomen and a small microphone-like instrument is moved around her belly to pick up sound waves that will create an image on a screen.

A Computerized Tomography (CT) scan is an important way to actually see the ovarian cancer. The CT scan uses x-ray images taken from different angles to create many detailed cross-sectional images of your body. These images can help identify tumors that may be on the ovary or have spread to the liver or other organs and can also help identify enlarged lymph nodes. This machine looks somewhat like a front load washing machine but much bigger and open at both ends. You will lie on a narrow table that slides in

---

[11] American Cancer Society: www.cancer.org

and out of the scanning machine. The technician will tell you to lie still and will tell you to hold your breath at certain times. A CT scan will take approximately ½ hour to complete.

A Positron Emission Tomography (PET scan) is another imaging procedure and it is done in the same machine as the CT scan. The PET scan uses a radioactive tracer, (usually sugar glucose) to look for cancer. All cells in the body need sugar to survive and they take up the radioactive tracer. But because cancer cells are fast growing, they take up more sugar than normal cells. The PET scan provides a picture of where those cancer cells are located and these places light up, especially if they have traveled to the lymph nodes or other parts of the body.

4) Biopsy

A biopsy is the removal of a sample of tissue to determine if the cells are cancerous. The cells are sent to the laboratory and examined by a pathologist under the microscope. In some cases, a needle biopsy can be done, for example, into an enlarged lymph node or into the abdomen if there is fluid build-up called ascites. For ovarian cancer, the tissue examination occurs during surgery when the tumor is removed. This is the essential step in reaching a diagnosis and provides information on the nature of the cells in terms of which subtype of ovarian cancer is present and which grade. This information is needed to guide further treatment with chemotherapy.

What about staging at diagnosis?[12]

Staging is the process of determining how far the cancer has spread. It is an important indicator of prognosis but also of how the cancer should be treated. Staging is based on three factors: 1) the extent and size of the tumor (T), 2) the spread to lymph nodes (N), and 3) the extent of metastasis (M). Staging requires a careful evaluation of each of these factors. In addition to the stage number, there are letters assigned, for example 1A, 1B, and 1C. Higher numbers means the cancer is more advanced as does higher letters.

Stage 1 includes those ovarian tumors in one or both ovaries but it has not spread to nearby lymph nodes or distant sites (metastasis). But in stage 1, there may be no cancer cells in the fluid in the abdomen and that would be classified as stages 1A and 1B. In Stage 1C there may be cancer cells in the abdominal fluid as well.

Stage II cancer has spread to local organs but not to the lymph nodes or to distant sites. In the abdomen, the spread could include the bladder, the uterus, the sigmoid colon or the rectum. Depending on these factors it will be classified as stage IIA or IIB.

Stage III cancer has spread to other organs in the pelvis or to the peritoneum lining and may have spread to abdominal lymph nodes. Depending on where it has spread in the abdomen and whether the lymph nodes locally (retroperitoneal lymph nodes) are involved it will be classified from IIIA to IIIC.

Stage IV disease has spread out of the abdomen. In stage IVA, cancer may be found in the fluid around the lungs but not on the liver, spleen, or lymph nodes outside the abdomen. In stage IVB the cancer has spread to the spleen or liver or to lymph nodes or other organs outside the abdominal peritoneal cavity including to the lungs or bones.

---

[12] Ovarian Cancer Research Alliance; www.ocrahope.org

What About Treatment ?[13]

The treatment plan will be based on the type of ovarian cancer, the grade, and the stage. Treatment for ovarian cancer will generally include surgery and chemotherapy and possibly other medications. Chemotherapy may be given before or after surgery and sometimes it is given both before and after surgery. When it is given before surgery it is called neoadjuvant chemotherapy. All of these decisions are made for each individual based on type, grade and stage.

Surgery: The objective of surgery is to remove all visible tumor whether confined to the ovaries or whether it has spread to adjacent organs. In most cases the ovaries, fallopian tubes, uterus, and omentum are all removed. In some cases where the disease has spread, additional organs such as the spleen and part of the bowel may also be removed. Removal of all visible tumor has been shown to be an important predictor of survival and it is necessary to find an experienced gynecological oncology surgeon to do this surgery.

Chemotherapy: The objective of chemotherapy is to kill cancer cells wherever they may be. For many years, the chemotherapy treatment has been carboplatin and a taxane. In more recent years, newer drugs have been developed including anti-angiogenesis drugs such as bevasizumab. Newly developed PARP inhibitors appear to be particularly effective for women with the BRCA1/2 mutations but are now also being used for women without these mutations. In some cases, these drugs might be given in conjunction with the initial standard chemotherapy and in some cases, they are given sequentially. Development of new therapies is ongoing and the availability of new drugs for ovarian cancer has increased in recent years and will continue to change and expand.

In addition to selecting the specific type of chemo, it can also be given in different ways. It can be given sequentially or concurrently, it can be given intravenously or intraperitoneal (through a port into the abdomen), and it can be given dose dense (weekly) or standard protocol (every three weeks.) There may be other options as well.

Unfortunately, immune therapy has not been found to be effective with ovarian cancer. There is a great deal of research on how to use an immune

---

[13] American Cancer Society: www.cancer.org

strategy to address ovarian cancer. Because it has been shown to be effective in other cancers, such as melanoma, many researchers are optimistic that eventually it will be developed to an effective treatment for ovarian cancer.

Treatment decisions are very complex and there is no way to adequately cover this topic here. The only way to know what is best for a particular woman is for her to work closely with a physician who specializes in ovarian cancer treatment, to select the optimal therapy for her circumstances, and to monitor the response.

What about treatment as part of clinical trials?[14]

Clinical trials are part of the research process of developing new therapies. When a new therapy is being developed, it is first tested in the lab and then it is tested with animals. The impact of the therapy and the side effects are examined. At some point, a promising new therapy needs to be tested in humans and that is where clinical trials are used. Clinical trials are research studies that enroll people.

A few notes regarding clinical trials:

Trials are available for all stages of cancer not just for people who have advanced or recurrent cancer.

There are two reasons for participating in a trial – to help yourself and to advance research so that women in the future will be helped as well.

Every trial is conducted by certain rules that are in place to protect patients and to assure the objectivity of the research.

There are three phases of clinical trials as new drugs progress from Phase 1, small numbers to test for safety, dosage, and efficacy, to Phase 3, large trials that give sufficient numbers to measure true efficacy, specify who might benefit, and identify side effects that may occur in small numbers of women.

Trials should not be regarded as options only after initial treatment has failed. While some trials require failures of initial treatment some trials take newly diagnosed patients. Trials are ways to test new drugs and trial participants will be the first to benefit from these drugs. Don't be afraid to discuss trials with your health care provider at any time during your treatment.

Every trial must have a plan called a "protocol" that explains how the trial will be run. You have a right to learn about the protocol and to have all of your questions answered before and while you are on the trial.

---

[14] American Cancer Society: www.cancer.org

It is up to the woman and her physician to determine if a trial is right for her. Anyone considering a trial has rights as a patient including learning about what drugs or treatments will be given and how, what medical tests will be done, who will cover costs if there are any, what the eligibility criteria are, and your rights to withdraw from the trial without penalty of any sort.

Not every medical center has access to every trial. If a trial is right for a particular woman, she may need to go to a more distant medical center to access the trial.

Treatments for ovarian cancer are improving because of these clinical trials. Trials are the major means of making progress on any disease. Resources that might help in making decisions about where to be treated and about what trials might be available can be found on the websites listed on the first page of the Appendix.

What you hear, what you say, how you feel, what you do.

When you are diagnosed with cancer, it feels like an earthquake in your life. Everything feels tossed around as though someone has taken a hold of your life and shaken it – nothing seems to be in the right place and some of your favorite possessions may have gotten smashed. You will be confused and scared and while the sirens are going off in your head, and you are at your worst, you will need to make sense of it all and figure out some of the most consequential choices you have ever faced. In the few pages here, I will share some information that might help you.

The most important reality is that you cannot run away from cancer. You cannot ignore it or pretend it isn't happening. You cannot pretend you don't need medical care. There are charlatans and alternative healers who may sound enticing but they are not going to help with your therapy. You cannot delay, procrastinate, or wish or pray for it to go away. There may be times that "fight or flight" can help save your life, but that is not the case with cancer. With cancer you are in for the long haul and you need to find the best care available.

The best care is available from those physicians and nurses who work with this disease every day, not just occasionally. If you love your general gynecologist that is great, but that doesn't mean this is the right person to treat your cancer. If your doctor has done lots of caesarian sections and hysterectomies, that does not qualify him or her to do surgery on your ovarian cancer. Almost every comprehensive cancer center will have a surgeon who sees patients with ovarian cancer every day and has the experience to perform this surgery. It is OK for you to ask for that person, it is OK for you to transfer doctors and hospitals. It may mean that you need to travel further than you want to for your surgery but that's worth it. All of the data show that women who have no visible disease at the end of surgery are more likely to survive. Because this disease can seed itself on other places in your abdomen, the surgeon needs to be able to find those places and remove what may be tiny start-up tumors. These are lengthy surgeries and it takes time and experience to get the best results.

At some hospitals, the surgeons also take charge of chemotherapy. This does not happen with most cancers. For example, the breast surgeon rarely does the chemotherapy for breast cancer. However, for ovarian cancer, this does happen. There seems to be a historical reason for this in that, as a rare cancer, there were few medical oncologists (the ones who administer chemo) who specialized in ovarian cancer. But that is changing now. There are physicians who specialize in medical oncology specifically for patients with ovarian cancer. This is important because this will be their primary interest and they may also be conducting research to advance the chemotherapy, immunotherapy and other treatments that may lead to the breakthroughs for this disease. So, you may be in a setting where the surgeon is in charge of the chemo or it may be a medical oncologist. Either can be prepared to help you make the best decisions about your therapy. Most important, though, is to find a doctor who specializes in ovarian cancer.

Ovarian cancer is a complex disease. You should get a second opinion from a second pathologist to determine that your tumor has been correctly diagnosed and typed. You can also get a second opinion about the therapy that will be prescribed for your cancer. You have a right to this and no physician should discourage you from doing this. However, you will need to resist the urge to shop around for a physician who tells you what you want to hear. Time is a factor with cancer and you need to get your first and second opinions quickly. You can help to expedite this by getting copies of your scans on discs (CDs)or on a flash drive so that you can take them with you to the second opinion consultation. CT scans are now often available on electronic medical systems and can be viewed by doctors at another hospital. You can also take tissue slides for a second pathology review.

Once you have decided on where you will be treated, you need to develop good relationships with your care team. You may feel angry. You may feel afraid. You may feel confused and distrustful. Still, it is important that you see your care team as there to help you and the relationship with your care team needs to be open and positive. And remember, you are the most important person on that team. You need to see yourself as part of a team where everyone is working to help you get better.

Continuity is important in care, and treatment is easier if you have the same care team all the way through. If your hospital makes it possible for you to do that, then don't feel bad asking for your favorite nurse for every infusion. I had infusions from three different nurses but if my favorite nurse was available, I always asked for her and that request was always honored. Don't be afraid to ask for the nurse you are most comfortable with.

While most side effects are predictable and expected, occasionally people experience side effects that are dangerous. You need to know who to call and when to call. You need to know when to call if you spike a fever, experience pain, experience mental confusion, have unrelenting vomiting or otherwise seem to be reacting badly after surgery or chemo. Ask for the physician to give you guidelines, write them down, share them with whoever may be helping you with your care, and don't delay if you experience any of these warning side effects.

Keep a log of your visits. Write the questions you have and the answers in your log. Take it with you every time you see your physician. You may have access to an electronic medical record that might be useful. But as I noted earlier, I have logged every CA-125 result for the past 10 years. They are written simply on a page of my log with the date noted. If I had had other side effects such a low platelets or anemia, I would have logged that as well. If I had had high blood pressure, I would have logged that also. The bottom line - take notes. You cannot remember everything that will take place during your treatment, but if you write it down during your visits in a small notebook, you can help monitor your care.

In line with this, write down your problems and questions and take them to your visits and ask for answers. This is not intrusive and if you are specific about your concerns the physician is more likely to be specific in answering your questions. Write down the answers as well. If there are words you don't understand, ask for an explanation. You are not expected to know medical terms but usually these can be explained in a way that you can understand. If you still don't understand then write it down and look up any terms after your visit.

Many studies have shown that coaching patients to write down questions and answers improves the visit satisfaction and increases patient understanding. Patient visits in a busy oncology clinic may be shorter than either the physician or the patient would prefer. For that reason, it helps if you can be efficient in your questioning.

Sometimes when people hear the word "cancer" what they really hear is the word "death". Because of this they often don't hear anything else after that word. It can help to have another person with you at your visits to help you with note taking and to help hear more clearly what the physician is saying. Your emotions can get in the way of hearing and you need to train yourself to listen carefully. This is especially important as the medical system allots less and less time to medical visits — a frustration to doctors and patients alike.

Hopefully what I have shared of my experiences will provide you with some suggestions on how to get through your diagnosis and treatment. Every person will have a different path, even though the central core of the surgery and chemo will be much the same. We all bring a different background, different experience of the disease, different strengths and weaknesses to the demands of the disease. Whatever works for you, whether it is meditation, walking, prayer, socializing, work, pets, solitude, sleeping – whatever brings you to a place of peace will be a good thing. Having said that, I have a few suggestions. It is important to balance unpleasant events with pleasant times even during treatment. Don't abandon everything that makes you happy while you are on chemo. You will need to get over any embarrassment regarding hair loss, slow walking, mental confusion or whatever else and continue to live your life, finding ways to enjoy and engage in whatever was meaningful to you before cancer.

There are many quotes about just "showing up." I suspect there are many times you experienced the worth of just showing up for work, for your volunteer efforts, and for your friends and family. With cancer, you need to just show up for yourself. Sometimes, women especially have a hard time just showing up for themselves. But with cancer, this is the time to show up for yourself, to value yourself enough to go through a rough time and believe you deserve to be cared for and respected for what you are doing. Only by showing up can you get optimal care. If you don't show up, if you drop out for a while or entirely, you won't get the best benefit of the therapy that is available.

And finally, it is important to take care of yourself. You need to eat good foods to the extent you can, you need to exercise to the extent you can and walking and stretching are sufficient. You need to take care of any part of your body that seems to be taking the brunt of the treatment whether it's your skin, your mouth, your digestive system, your bone marrow, or your mind. You need to do whatever you can to get through and because your care team has seen it all before, they can help you figure it out if you ask. And you need to know that your body has an amazing ability to recover.

Keeping your emotions and mental state calm and resilient is as important as taking care of your body. Many women find comfort in support groups with other women going through a cancer diagnosis even if it is a different form of cancer. These groups may allow you to say what lays heavy on your heart without fear of upsetting family or friends or worse, having them respond in ways that are not helpful. If your hospital does not have a support group, you might contact the Ovarian Cancer Research Alliance (OCRA), American Cancer Society, FORCE, Gilda's club, the Wellness community or the ovarian cancer support organizations in your community. (Gilda's club is named after Gilda Radner, a Saturday

Night Live comedian who died of ovarian cancer. If you don't know who she was — just google her and enjoy a laugh.)

You may find that church or prayer are helpful. You may find that you just need family and friends. You may find just getting outside is helpful. You may find that meditation or yoga or exercise help you. You are free to distance yourself from people and places that are not helpful and cling to those that are. Don't feel guilty if that is the case, the priority must be on yourself right now. There are people who will help you. Most often these are people who have been important to you for a very long time. Sometimes these are unexpected angels and might even be someone you never knew before your diagnosis. So, be open to meeting new people who may come to your side and help you. Without being insensitive to others, you need to be somewhat selfish in taking care of yourself. This is the time to put yourself first.

To anyone newly diagnosed or living with this disease, I hope that sharing my experience and thoughts in this book will be helpful to you. I wish you the very best.

ACKNOWLEDGEMENTS

The fact that I am here to tell this story is due to the extraordinary health care and kindness of my medical team: Agustin Garcia MD, Laila Muderspach, MD, Darcy Spicer MD, Sue Ellen Martin MD, Mabel Vasquez MD, Lilia Frausto RN NP, Laurie Feinstein RN and Imelda Solomon RN. I hope I have done justice to communicating what optimal health care looks like and feels like. This level of health care needs to be a standard for women with ovarian cancer. Correct that — this level of health care needs to be a standard.

And with great thanks to those who sat with me through many days hooked up to the chemo infusion pump. First my husband Jim Richardson and my friends Susan Groshen, Sue Stoyanoff, Kay Johnson, Sue Ellen Martin, Yvonne Barranday, Lourdes Baezconde-Garbanati, Don Feinstein, and Kathleen Dwyer. And thanks to those friends and family who called, and visited, and helped me in ways too many to mention and to those who prayed.

And to the faculty and staff of the Department of Preventive Medicine who supported me and picked up my responsibilities during the hard days of treatment and recovery.

And to Maggie and Juliann who got us back outside camping and hiking and to Alexandra for our walk-talks from before this all began and on to today.

The fact that this book got written is due to the encouragement and feedback from Jim Richardson, Barbara Abercrombie, Alexandra Levine, Mary Aalto, Donald Miller, Darcy Spicer, Agustin Garcia, Andy Berchuck, Barry LeCerf, Margi Denton and my amazing writing group, Michelle Peterson, Lauren Tyler-Rickon, Lena Nelson, Anne Witzgall, Valerie Silverio, Jim Garbanati, and Marilyn Davis.

Most of all, I am grateful for the love of my family and the joy that they bring to my life: Jim, Katherine and Mike, David and Ali, and the grandchildren Thomas, Connor, Trevor, Ryan, Eden and Chase.

Jean LeCerf Richardson

Made in USA - Kendallville, IN
64157_9780578358925
01.20.2022 0854